Understanding the
Menopause
and HRT

Professor Anne MacGregor

Published by Family Doctor Publications Limited
in association with the British Medical Association

IMPORTANT

This book is intended not as a substitute for personal medical advice but as a supplement to that advice for the patient who wishes to understand more about his or her condition.

Before taking any form of treatment
YOU SHOULD ALWAYS CONSULT YOUR MEDICAL PRACTITIONER.

In particular (without limit) you should note that advances in medical science occur rapidly and some information about drugs and treatment contained in this booklet may very soon be out of date.

Family Doctor Publications, PO Box 4664, Poole, Dorset BH15 1NN

ISBN-13: 978 1 903474 24 2
ISBN-10: 1 903474 24 8

20052013

Contents

The menopause: what happens to
your body? 1

Helping yourself feel better 14

Replacing the hormones (HRT) 35

The benefits of HRT 45

The risks of HRT 61

Different types of HRT 75

How to take HRT 97

HRT: when to start and when to stop 104

Side effects of HRT 108

HRT: who can and who can't take it 117

Controlling symptoms without HRT 123

Contraception around the menopause 129

HRT: conclusions 137

Questions and answers 140

Glossary 148

Useful addresses 154

Index 163

Your pages 177

About the author

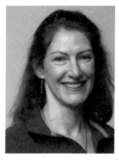

Professor Anne MacGregor is a specialist in headache and women's health, Barts Health NHS Trust, and is an instructing doctor for the Faculty of Sexual and Reproductive Healthcare of The Royal College of Obstetricians and Gynaecologists.

The menopause: what happens to your body?

What is the 'menopause'?

The word 'menopause' strictly means a woman's last menstrual period, which typically occurs around the age of 51, and defines the end of the fertile phase of a woman's life. The 'change of life' or 'climacteric' is the time when your body is adjusting before, during and after the menopause. There are hormonal changes and symptoms in the years leading up to, and beyond, your final menstrual period. It has been estimated that, by the age of 54 years, most women (80 per cent) have had their last menstrual period – they are then termed postmenopausal.

Some women experience a natural menopause before the age of 40. This is considered premature. Menopause can be induced prematurely by radiotherapy or chemotherapy used to treat some cancers, or following surgery to remove the ovaries. In such women, hot flushes and sweats can be particularly severe.

The menstrual cycle

Every month between puberty and the menopause, a mature egg is released and the lining of the uterus becomes thicker, ready for a fertilised egg to implant. If the egg is not fertilised it passes out of the body during menstruation.

1. The principal changes in hormones during the menstrual cycle

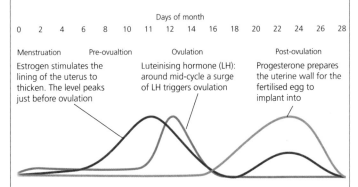

Days of month

0   2   4   6   8   10   11   12   14   16   18   20   22   24   26   28

Menstruation   Pre-ovualtion   Ovulation   Post-ovulation

Estrogen stimulates the lining of the uterus to thicken. The level peaks just before ovulation

Luteinising hormone (LH): around mid-cycle a surge of LH triggers ovulation

Progesterone prepares the uterine wall for the fertilised egg to implant into

2. Changes in the lining of the uterus during the menstrual cycle

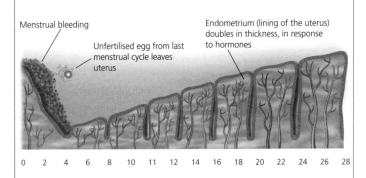

Menstrual bleeding

Unfertilised egg from last menstrual cycle leaves uterus

Endometrium (lining of the uterus) doubles in thickness, in response to hormones

0   2   4   6   8   10   11   12   14   16   18   20   22   24   26   28

The change in estrogen levels over a lifetime

Until the menopause, women produce estrogen in varying amounts over a 28-day cycle. However, after the menopause, estrogen production falls to a low level and this increases the risk of bone fractures, strokes and heart disease.

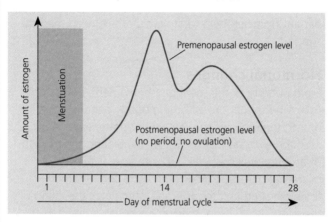

Estrogen levels gradually decline towards the menopause. After the menopause the ovaries cease functioning, estrogen levels fall and periods stop.

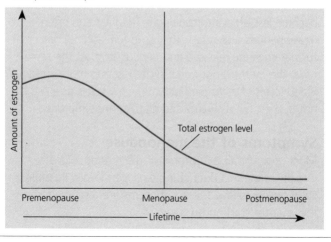

Many women adjust to the changes without problems and some revel in their new-found freedom – free from the monthly 'curse' of periods, particularly if periods were painful or heavy, and free from the fear of unwanted pregnancy. However, not all women find the change of life easy and, although some may benefit from self-help treatments, others need medical support.

Hormonal changes

From puberty to the menopause, women's bodies follow hormonal cycles – the monthly periods. Each month the levels of the female hormone, estrogen, rise over the early part of the cycle, stimulating the growth of an egg, which is released from one of the two ovaries at mid-cycle. Following ovulation, another female hormone, progesterone, stimulates the lining of the uterus to thicken, ready for a possible pregnancy. If the egg is not fertilised by a sperm, it dies and the egg and uterus lining are shed as a period.

In the years leading up to the menopause, the ovaries become less efficient, resulting in irregular and often heavy periods. Eventually, they stop functioning, no further eggs are released and periods stop. At the same time, the monthly hormonal cycle becomes more erratic. Blood levels of estrogen fluctuate – low levels give rise to hot flushes, night sweats and many other symptoms.

Symptoms of the menopause

Most, but not all, symptoms of the menopause are directly related to fluctuating estrogen levels. Possible solutions to relieve these symptoms are discussed in the chapter starting on page 14.

Irregular periods

This is usually the first sign that signals the menopause. As the ovaries become erratic in their production of estrogen and progesterone, so your menstrual cycle becomes irregular. At first your cycle typically shortens from its usual 28 days to between 21 and 25 days. Later on, it lengthens, with occasional skipped periods. Your period itself can change – sometimes it may be very heavy and last longer than usual, at other times it may be scanty and short. Fewer cycles result in the release of an egg and so you become less fertile. Sometimes an egg is spontaneously released following an apparent menopause, so you should use adequate contraception until a year or two after your final period.

Hot flushes and night sweats

Hot flushes and night sweats are hallmark symptoms of the menopause, affecting about 75 per cent of women.

Flushes often start around the age of 47 or 48 and usually continue for three or four years. In the early stages of the menopause they may occur only in the week before menstruation, when estrogen levels are naturally low. Eventually, estrogen levels fluctuate sufficiently throughout the cycle so that flushes happen at any time. Flushes reach their peak during the first couple of years after the last menstrual period, and then ease over time.

In some women flushes start earlier; for some it happens in their late 30s or early 40s. Flushes can continue for 5 or 10 years; 25 per cent of women will have occasional flushes for more than 5 years. A Swedish study found that about 9 per cent of 72-year-old women have hot flushes.

Symptoms of the menopause

There are many symptoms associated with the menopause, mainly caused by changes in the levels of estrogen in the body. Fortunately, most women do not suffer from all the symptoms.

- Anxiety
- Changes to skin and hair
- Depression
- Disrupted sleep
- Dry vagina
- Fatigue
- Headaches
- Hot flushes and night sweats
- Irregular periods
- Irritability
- Joint and muscle pain
- Loss of interest in sex
- Painful intercourse
- Palpitations of the heart
- Poor concentration
- Poor memory
- Urinary problems

Many women can sense when a flush is about to start, often noticing a feeling of increasing pressure in the head and a faster pulse. Within a few minutes, the flush rapidly spreads across the shoulders and chest, rising up the neck and head. This often causes great discomfort and embarrassment. Flushes usually last a matter of seconds but can persist for 15 minutes or so, recurring several times during the day. You might also notice sweating or palpitations and feel weak or faint. Night sweats can be particularly severe, disrupting sleep – some women have to change their night-clothes and even their sheets because they wake drenched in sweat.

Disrupted sleep

Symptoms such as night sweats are not the only reason for disrupted sleep. Such symptoms can also be a symptom of underlying anxiety or depression. Anxiety usually causes difficulty getting to sleep – you feel extremely tired but your mind keeps ticking over the events of the day or you worry about the future. Depression is more often associated with early morning waking – you get to sleep without too much trouble but wake in the early hours tossing and turning until it is time to get up.

As the hormonal changes of the menopause can aggravate underlying anxiety and depression, specific medical treatment for these conditions may be necessary. So, if sleepless nights continue, particularly if you have successfully controlled other symptoms of the 'change', you should seek help from your doctor.

Headaches

Fluctuating hormone levels can trigger migraine and other headaches in susceptible women. During the 'change' women notice an increasing link between headaches and their monthly periods. Premenstrual symptoms, that is, occurring a week or two before a period, become more prominent at this time of life and both migraine and non-migraine headaches can worsen during the premenstrual week. Headaches usually improve when hormonal fluctuations settle after the menopause. If the headaches are troublesome, your doctor or a specialist headache clinic can advise on specific treatment.

Joint and muscle pains

Aching wrists, knees and ankles, and lower back pain are common and may often be confused with arthritis.

Painful intercourse

Estrogen stimulates the production of mucus, which keeps the vagina and other sexual parts moist. After the menopause, lack of estrogen means that less lubricating mucus is produced. The vagina becomes shorter, less elastic and dryer. As well as intercourse becoming more painful, these changes can result in itching and irritation. However, sexual excitement stimulates the production of lubricating fluids, so prolonged foreplay can help prevent painful intercourse.

Loss of libido

Sexual desire frequently lessens with the menopause and it often takes longer to become aroused. Sexual desire is also affected by general well-being, emotional upsets and painful intercourse.

Urinary symptoms

A sudden need to urinate (urge incontinence), even when you have just been to the toilet, is a common problem after the menopause; lack of estrogen causes the tissues around the neck of the bladder to thin. Also the muscles that support the uterus and prevent the bladder from leaking become weaker.

Coughing and running typically provoke an embarrassing leak of urine (stress incontinence), which affects between 10 and 20 per cent of women over 60 and up to 40 per cent of women in their 80s. Stress incontinence also commonly affects women in their late 40s and throughout their 50s.

Recurring urine infections are also more common as the skin around the bladder becomes thinner and drier. Estrogen deficiency changes the acidity of the vaginal secretions, resulting in fewer of the protective bacteria being present that help to fight off infection before the menopause. A common sign of possible infection is burning or stinging when urinating.

Dry skin and hair

Estrogen keeps your skin moist and stimulates hair growth – hence the 'bloom' of pregnancy when estrogen levels are very high. Without estrogen your skin becomes dry, losing its suppleness so that wrinkles become more prominent. Hair growth slows but the rate of hair loss stays the same so your hair becomes thinner and less manageable.

Dry eyes

As well as skin becoming drier after the menopause, many women notice that their eyes become persistently dry and itchy as fewer tears are produced.

Weight gain

Women may put on weight because of reduced physical activity – perhaps just as a result of lifestyle changes but maybe because of joint problems. As we age our bodies burn up energy more slowly than when we were younger, which can also lead to weight gain if we don't either eat less or exercise more. Hormonal changes also play a role, because estrogen is responsible for maintaining the female shape; after the menopause weight tends to settle more around the waist than the hips.

Emotional symptoms

Poor sleep has a knock-on effect resulting in daytime tiredness, lethargy, difficulty concentrating and depression. These symptoms are often very distressing and make it even harder to cope with daily demands. Finding ways to improve sleep, either by controlling the flushes or by treating depression, can help restore the balance.

Non-hormonal symptoms

Depression and sexual problems around the menopause are not just the result of falling levels of estrogen. The menopause marks a time in a woman's life that can be difficult for many reasons – it may coincide with children leaving home, impending retirement, marital difficulties, ill or dying parents. These changes take their own toll and may need professional support. Some women may benefit from professional support which is available through GPs.

Diagnosing the 'change'

The symptoms of the 'change' are usually sufficient evidence to make the diagnosis, particularly for women in their late 40s or early 50s. If there is any uncertainty about the diagnosis, for example if a woman experiences an unusually early menopause, the diagnosis can be confirmed by a simple blood test to check the hormone levels. Unless a woman's periods have stopped completely, the blood tests are usually taken within the first week of the menstrual cycle, the first day of the cycle being the first day of bleeding. These tests check the levels of follicle-stimulating homone (FSH) and luteinising hormone (LH), which are higher than usual if a woman is perimenopausal (close to the menopause). Sometimes a second test is taken about a week before the expected start of menstruation to measure the levels of progesterone. The presence of this hormone confirms that the woman has ovulated that cycle. As these blood tests give a result only for

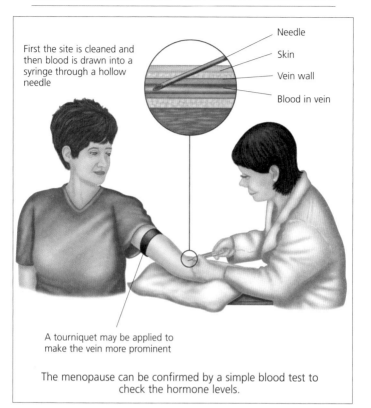

First the site is cleaned and then blood is drawn into a syringe through a hollow needle

Needle

Skin

Vein wall

Blood in vein

A tourniquet may be applied to make the vein more prominent

The menopause can be confirmed by a simple blood test to check the hormone levels.

that particular menstrual cycle, and normal hormone surges can occasionally confuse the results, the results must be viewed in the context of all the symptoms – a single normal result does not exclude the menopause.

Postmenopausal risks

The menopause has taken on much greater importance over recent years, particularly in western society, because, with a life expectancy of over 80 years (and rising), many women can expect to be postmenopausal for over one-third of their lives.

Although the symptoms of the menopause are not life threatening, the long-term effects of estrogen deficiency can be. The major diseases of old age are heart disease, strokes, breast and bowel cancer, osteoporosis and fractures, and dementia. All of these are affected by estrogen so women with a premature menopause are at particular risk. Although these conditions do not always result in death, they may lead to a significant reduction in quality of life, for both the individuals affected and their relatives.

KEY POINTS

■ There are many symptoms of the 'change' and they vary from mild to severe

■ Typical symptoms are irregular periods, hot flushes and night sweats

■ Symptoms can also include mood changes, difficulty sleeping and depression

■ Diagnosis of the menopause is usually based on the symptoms

■ Most symptoms settle within a few years of periods stopping

■ Women now live longer and the long-term effects of estrogen deficiency are increasingly apparent; the risk of fractures, strokes and heart disease increases with each year after the menopause

Helping yourself feel better

Menopausal symptoms

Simple measures are worth trying before complementary or prescription therapies are considered, particularly if the symptoms are relatively mild.

Flushes and sweats

Keep cool – hot flushes can be triggered by a rise in temperature, eating hot spicy foods, or hot drinks such as tea or coffee. Anecdotally, women report that using a fan and drinking cold drinks can help. Wear natural fibres that allow air to circulate around the skin and layer thinner clothes rather than wearing one thick sweater. Use cotton sheets or duvet covers and sleep in a cool room with adequate ventilation.

Exercise

Physically active women experience fewer and less severe flushes than sedentary women.

Lose weight
A high body mass (being overweight) predisposes to more frequent and severe flushes.

Stop smoking
The more a woman smokes, the more flushes she is likely to have.

Relax
Slow, controlled breathing can reduce the severity of a flush when performed as soon as a flush begins.

Disrupted sleep
The above strategies of exercise, weight loss and relaxation similarly apply to improving sleep. Avoid stimulating food and drink near bedtime, particularly alcohol – try a warm milky drink instead. Have a warm bath and read a book or watch TV until you feel sleepy, but beware of thrillers and other stimulating programmes! Keep the room cool with circulating fresh air. If you wake in the night and cannot go back to sleep, get up, make a drink and read for a while. If you feel tired during the day, take a 20-minute nap – longer than this will make it harder to sleep at night.

Irregular periods
As periods become more irregular, they often also become heavier and more painful. Mild period problems can be helped by gentle exercise or heat but heavy, painful periods often require specific treatment. If simple painkillers don't help, visit the doctor for advice. As heavy periods can lead to anaemia, boost iron intake with iron-rich foods such as meat and spinach, or with iron supplements.

Headaches

Most headaches result from some obvious underlying cause such as missed meals, lack of sleep or muscular pain. Migraine headaches can arise from similar triggers so help reduce frequent attacks by eating regularly and getting enough sleep. Simple painkillers or over-the-counter migraine treatments help to control symptoms but follow the instructions and do not take them for more than a couple of days a week; more frequent use can exacerbate the problem as rebound symptoms occur. Also, frequent use of painkillers can suppress the body's own natural painkillers, the endorphins, increasing pain. If headaches do not respond to simple measures, see a doctor who can advise on treatment, including drugs to treat and to prevent attacks. For more information on headaches see the Family Doctor book *Understanding Migraine and Other Headaches*.

Joint and muscle pains

Deep-heat creams and gels or a heat-pad can give some relief but painkillers, such as paracetamol, or anti-inflammatory drugs, such as aspirin or ibuprofen, may be necessary if your symptoms are severe. If these are not effective, seek the advice of a general practitioner. Try gentle, non-weight-bearing exercise such as cycling or swimming. Losing weight can reduce the load on your joints. Fish oil supplements and glucosamine may help.

Vaginal dryness

If vaginal dryness is the only problem, lubricating gels may help. They can be bought from a pharmacy. Never use petroleum jelly, or other oil-based products, because these prevent air reaching the skin and increase the risk of infections. Smear the product liberally over the vulval area, particularly round the opening of the vagina. Replens and Senselle are artificial lubricants that are used two or three times a week. They coat the inside of the vagina with a non-hormonal moisturiser, which lasts for a day or two, so they do not have to be used immediately before intercourse. In contrast, KY jelly needs to be used just before intercourse.

Loss of libido

Sex drive naturally lessens over the years and it takes longer to get aroused. Whereas younger women may become sufficiently aroused for penetrative sex in as short a time as a few seconds, menopausal women may take five minutes or more. Taking time during sex, with lots of foreplay, enables the Bartholin's glands to produce the maximum amount of lubrication before penetration.

Urinary symptoms

Simply crossing the legs when you feel a cough or sneeze starting can help prevent leakage. Eat plenty of fresh fruit, vegetables and fibre to avoid constipation, which can cause pressure on the bladder and urethra.

Strengthening the pelvic floor muscles

Also try to lose weight, because being overweight puts stress on the pelvic floor muscles. These muscles provide support to the bladder, rectum and uterus. They are weakened by childbirth and are further weakened by estrogen deficiency after the menopause. Strengthening the muscles can help reduce leakage.

The most common technique is pelvic floor exercises, sometimes known as Kegel exercises after their inventor Dr Arnold Kegel. You may have to do them for a few months before you notice any improvement. You can do them at any time – while driving the car, doing the housework, talking on the phone.

Sit with your knees slightly apart and imagine that you are trying to stop yourself passing wind from the back passage; to do this you must tighten the muscles round your back passage. Squeeze and lift those muscles as if you really do have wind: you should be able to feel the muscles move and the skin round the back passage tightening. Your legs and buttocks should not move at all.

Then imagine that you are sitting on the toilet urinating. Imagine yourself trying to stop the stream of urine. Hold the muscles tight for at least five seconds if you can, then relax.

Repeat at least five times. Now pull the muscles up quickly and tightly. Repeat at least five times. Do these exercises – five slow and five fast – at least ten times every day.

Small weighted plastic cones inserted into the vagina, which can be bought from the chemist, can help exercise the correct muscles, because the pelvic floor muscles have to be tensed to prevent the cones falling out.

If you find these exercises difficult or ineffective, your doctor can give advice or may refer you to a specialist continence adviser.

Urinary infections

Do not restrict the amount of fluids that you drink as this can worsen the problem by increasing your susceptibility to cystitis because harmful bacteria are

Strengthening bladder control

1. Pelvic floor exercises involve consciously contracting the muscles that support the uterus, bowel and bladder, in order to strengthen them. This brings greater control of the bladder and can help to reduce incontinence.

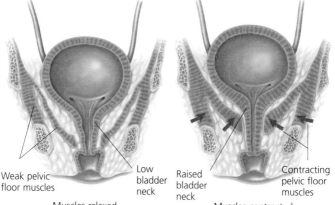

Weak pelvic floor muscles

Low bladder neck

Muscles relaxed

Raised bladder neck

Contracting pelvic floor muscles

Muscles contracted

2. Placing a weighted plastic cone in the vagina and contracting the pelvic floor muscles to keep it there can help to develop the muscles that control the bladder.

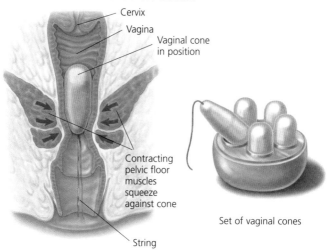

Cervix

Vagina

Vaginal cone in position

Contracting pelvic floor muscles squeeze against cone

String

Set of vaginal cones

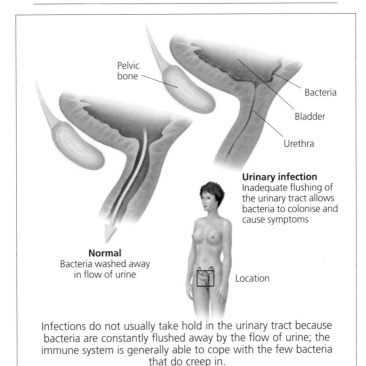

Urinary infection
Inadequate flushing of the urinary tract allows bacteria to colonise and cause symptoms

Normal
Bacteria washed away in flow of urine

Location

Infections do not usually take hold in the urinary tract because bacteria are constantly flushed away by the flow of urine; the immune system is generally able to cope with the few bacteria that do creep in.

less likely to be urinated away. But do cut out coffee, strong tea and other caffeine-rich drinks, such as fizzy cola, that stimulate the bladder muscle.

Cystitis may respond to treatments from the chemist containing sodium citrate, which makes the urine less acidic. Alternatively, drink cranberry juice or water with a teaspoon of bicarbonate of soda added which also makes the urine less acidic. If your symptoms do not ease within a day or so, see your doctor as you may have an infection and need antibiotics.

Dry skin and hair
Keep to a simple haircut that is easy to manage and use

conditioner to stop your hair becoming too dry. If you are out in the sun, use an effective sun cream and wear a hat. If you swim regularly, wear a swimming hat and apply plenty of moisturiser after showering, as chlorine is very drying to both skin and hair.

Dry eyes

Women frequently experience problems with dry eyes as they enter the menopause. Many find relief simply from using artificial tears that can be bought from a pharmacy. There are a variety of different chemicals used, including hypromellose, hydroxyethylcellulose, liquid paraffin or saline solution. Preservative-free tears are the most soothing. Avoid products that whiten the eyes – they do not have adequate lubricating qualities and often make the problem worse. Simple lifestyle changes can significantly improve irritation from dry eyes; for example, drinking eight to ten glasses of water spaced over the course of each day keeps the body hydrated. Make a conscious effort to blink frequently – especially when reading, working at the computer or watching television. Avoid rubbing the eyes as it only worsens the irritation.

If simple remedies are not effective, see a doctor – certain medications, thyroid conditions, vitamin A deficiency and diseases such as Parkinson's disease and Sjögren's syndrome, a condition where the immune system attacks the glands that produce tears and saliva, can also cause dryness.

Weight gain

Increasing evidence suggests that postmenopausal weight gain is nature's way of producing more estrogen. After the menopause a certain amount of estrogen is formed in fat, so the fatter you are, the more estrogen you produce. This may explain why, in general, fat women have stronger bones than thin women. Obviously, a balance is necessary because obesity is linked to heart disease. The simple message is that, in most cases, keeping fit and eating a healthy balanced diet allow weight to settle at its natural level.

Emotional symptoms

Most of us have felt low at some time in our lives. Usually it is the result of a particular event, and these feelings eventually ease with time. Hormonal changes can make it harder to cope. Finding ways to relax and unwind, eating healthily and taking adequate exercise will all improve mood. Limit consumption of alcohol because it can aggravate depression. Seek medical help early – a supportive doctor may be all that is needed, but counselling or drug therapy may be necessary.

Preventing heart disease and osteoporosis
What is heart disease?

The heart is essentially a muscle that pumps blood around the body. Blood vessels, or arteries, supply blood to the heart muscle. When blood flow through the arteries becomes obstructed, the heart muscle can die – this is when a heart attack occurs. The most common way such obstructions develop is through a condition called atherosclerosis, a largely preventable disease. Blood vessels to the brain can also be affected by atherosclerosis, which can result in strokes.

Lifestyle changes to prevent heart disease

Many of the risk factors for heart disease can be reduced

by simple lifestyle changes: losing weight, stopping smoking, modifying diet and taking more exercise.

What is osteoporosis?

Osteoporosis is a disease in which bones become fragile and more likely to break. Unfortunately there are no symptoms of osteoporosis until a bone breaks. These broken bones, known as fractures, typically affect the hip, spine and wrist.

A hip fracture can cause prolonged or permanent disability or even death. Spinal or vertebral fractures also have serious consequences, including loss of height, severe back pain and deformity.

Lifestyle changes to prevent osteoporosis

Adequate exercise and a healthy calcium-rich diet keep bones strong. Effective prevention of osteoporosis starts early, however, preferably in childhood – there is plenty that can be done to protect children. They need exercise and a good diet including calcium-rich foods, and should be warned about the hazards of smoking. Peak adult bone mass is reached around the age of 35. The peak bone mass for men is 25 to 30 per cent greater than for women, placing women at greater risk of osteoporosis. Bone loss starts shortly after the peak, starting earlier in women than in men, and is accelerated by the menopause.

Exercise for a healthy heart and strong bones

The value of exercise cannot be overemphasised. Studies show that being physically fit lowers heart disease risk even in people who have other health problems such as high blood pressure and high cholesterol. To minimise risk, however, you should be

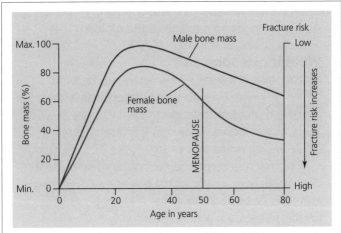

Bone mass peaks between the ages of 25 and 40 in men and women and then starts to fall. In women, accelerated loss of bone mass occurs around the time of the menopause.

physically fit and avoid the other major modifiable risk factors: cigarette smoke, high blood pressure and high blood cholesterol.

It is never too late to start exercising – one study showed that an 80 year old gains the same percentage improvement in muscle strength as a 25 year old. If you are inactive, doing anything is better than nothing! Studies show that people who have a low fitness level are much more likely to die earlier than people who have achieved even a moderate level of fitness. It is not just your heart and bones that benefit from regular exercise; muscle strength and power also improve, making falls less likely and, if you do trip, you have more strength to grab on to something. If you take drugs such as tranquillisers, hypnotics or alcohol, reassess your need for them as they may affect your judgement, making you more likely to trip or stumble.

Weight-bearing exercise strengthens bone and can also help to prevent fractures. The easiest and most convenient exercise is walking – which strengthens your heart and bones. Start gently and gradually increase the distance. Swimming is not weight bearing because the body is supported by the water, but it is excellent if you have joint problems and is also good for the heart.

Although the recommendation for exercise is 30 minutes a week, this need not be as daunting as it sounds as it can be made up of 1-minute bouts of brisk activities. Climbing, gardening, moderate-to-heavy housework, dancing and home exercise are all beneficial. Again, doing anything is better than nothing.

Middle-aged or older people who are inactive and at high risk for heart disease or who already have a medical condition should seek medical advice before starting or significantly increasing their physical activity.

Exercise as a daily routine

The main reason why people fail to take exercise is simply a lack of time to incorporate exercise into their daily routine. Why not walk or cycle to the shops instead of taking the bus or car; if it is too far, get off the bus one stop earlier, or park your car further away. If you feel up to more formal exercise, such as jogging, go ahead but be careful not to overdo it in the early stages.

Always warm up and cool down gradually to prevent injury to muscles. Avoid vigorous exercise if you are unwell because it can put an undue strain on your heart. Remember, an exercise programme should be maintained for life, not just for a few weeks a year.

Watch your diet
Natural estrogens
Some studies suggest that natural estrogens found in many plant foods, particularly beans and pulses, can protect against osteoporosis, heart disease and breast cancer. Certainly, the incidence of these diseases is much lower in countries such as Japan where estrogen-rich soya bean products, such as tofu, are an essential part of the diet.

Calcium
Bones contain calcium, so a healthy diet with adequate calcium is necessary to ensure that bones develop properly and remain strong. Periods of growth obviously increase the relative demands for calcium, so teenagers and pregnant women need greater amounts. The recommended daily amount for adults is 700 milligrams (mg). Dairy foods such as milk, cheese and yoghurt are the best sources of calcium, which is readily absorbed into the bloodstream. Unfortunately, the current fashion for dieting has meant that many women cut out dairy products because they also contain high levels of fat. The answer is to continue eating dairy products but switch to low-fat alternatives – skimmed milk actually contains slightly more calcium than whole milk. Tinned bony fish such as sardines or salmon is excellent because the softened bones are rich in calcium.

Vitamin D
This vitamin helps the absorption of calcium. Dietary intake of vitamin D has declined over the years and may be linked to increasing fracture rates. Fatty fish, such as halibut, mackerel and salmon, are rich sources of vitamin D; studies suggest that two meals of fatty

Dietary sources of calcium

Dairy products (average portion)	Calcium content (milligrams or mg)	Non-dairy products (average portion)	Calcium content (mg)
Skimmed milk: 190 millilitres (third of a pint)	235	Tofu (steamed): 100 g	510
Semi-skimmed milk: 190 ml (third of a pint)	231	Sardines in oil (drained): 60 g	220
Whole milk: 190 ml (third of a pint)	224	Dried figs: 30 g	75
Yoghurt: 140 g (5 oz)	240	Baked beans: 120 g (4 oz)	50
Edam cheese: 30 g (1 oz)	216	1 orange	47
Cheddar cheese: 30 g (1 oz)	207	1 slice of white bread	28
Cottage cheese: 30 g (1 oz)	82	1 slice of brown bread	7

fish a week can reduce the fracture risk by up to 20 per cent.

Supplementing your diet

Calcium supplements are a useful addition to a poor diet, particularly in early life when bones are developing. If you have been diagnosed with osteoporosis you will need to supplement your diet to ensure that you get around 1,000–1,200 mg of calcium daily. Vitamin D is also available as supplements of 400–800 international units or IU (10–20 micrograms) daily. It is often combined with calcium. Be careful not to overdo it, and try to meet your daily requirements through diet rather than supplements – taking more than 2,000 mg of calcium can increase your risk of kidney stones and may interfere with your absorption of other minerals such as iron.

Cut down on alcohol

Although moderate drinking is thought to be beneficial to health, heavy drinking increases your risk of osteoporosis and heart disease in addition to its effects on general health. The density of the hip bone is reduced by up to 12 per cent in women in their late 40s who regularly drink more than two units of alcohol

What is a unit of alcohol?
A one-litre bottle of spirits – brandy, whisky or gin – contains about 40 units of alcohol

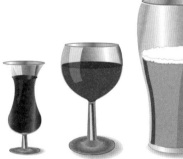
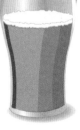

| A small glass of sherry or fortified wine | A standard glass of wine 1.5 units | ½ pint of beer or cider ¼ pint of strong lager | A single measure of aperitif or spirit |

a day, so try to drink no more than this. There is no need to go teetotal because a small amount of alcohol (one to two units a day) helps protect against heart disease and stroke. One unit of alcohol is equivalent to half a pint of beer, cider or lager (three to four per cent alcohol by volume), a small pub measure of spirits, or a standard pub measure of sherry or fortified wine. One and a half units of alcohol are equivalent to a small glass (125 millilitres) of ordinary strength wine or standard pub measure of spirits. Remember that stronger beers and wines will contain more units of alcohol.

Control your weight

Middle-aged spread can help maintain bone density, because hormones produced by the adrenal gland and the postmenopausal ovaries are converted to estrogen in fat cells. However, it is important to keep a healthy weight because being overweight is associated with increased risk of heart disease and strokes.

The body mass index (BMI) is a useful index of healthy weight and is easily calculated if you know your weight, measured in kilograms, and your height, measured in metres. The recommended BMI is between 18.5 and 24.9. If your BMI is less than 18.4, you are underweight for your height; if it is between 25 and 29.9, you are over the ideal weight for your height; if it is over 30, you are obese. To calculate your own BMI, divide your weight by the square of your height. For example, if you weigh 11 stone, that is approximately 70 kg. If you are 5 feet 6 inches tall, that is approximately 168 cm or 1.68 m. Your BMI is the square of your height $(1.68 \times 1.68 = 2.82)$ divided into your weight: $70/2.82 = 24.8$. So your BMI is approximately 24.8 (see page 30).

What should you weigh?

- The body mass index (BMI) is a useful measure of healthy weight
- Find out your height in metres and weight in kilograms
- Calculate your BMI like this:

$$BMI = \frac{Your\ weight\ (kg)}{[Your\ height\ (metres) \times Your\ height\ (metres)]}$$

$$e.g.\ 24.8 = \frac{70}{[1.68 \times 1.68]}$$

- You are recommended to try to maintain a BMI in the range 18.5–24.9
- The chart below is an easier way of estimating your BMI. Read off your height and your weight. The point where the lines cross in the chart indicates your BMI

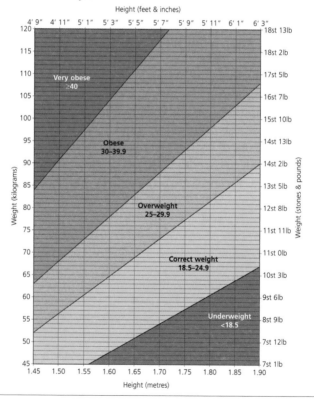

Height (feet & inches)

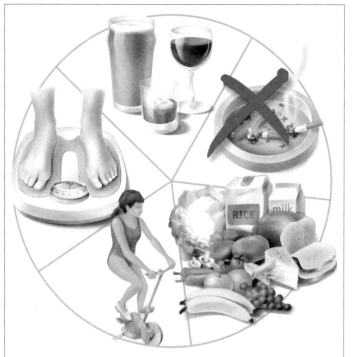

You can do a lot to help your long-term health by making simple lifestyle changes: maintain the correct weight for your height, stop smoking, drink alcohol in moderation, eat plenty of fruit, vegetables and food rich in calcium, and take regular exercise.

Stop smoking

Smoking increases the risk of heart disease, fractures and cancers. Women who smoke have a menopause one or two years earlier than non-smokers.

Complementary treatments

Many women are concerned about the effects of drugs on their bodies and are keen to find alternative ways to control their symptoms. Acupuncture, aromatherapy, biofeedback, herbalism, homoeopathy, osteopathy, physiotherapy and other treatments may be helpful but there is little research into the benefits and potential risks. It is important to go to qualified therapists. Further information can be obtained from the official organisations representing each of the specialties – see Useful addresses (page 154).

Keeping healthy
Breast self-awareness
Being aware of any changes in your breasts is very important. Every woman's breasts are different so it is much easier for her to identify any changes.

What is normal for one woman may not be for another. One woman's breasts will also look and feel different over time depending on the time of the month and the age of the woman. Learning how your breasts look and feel at different times will help you to know what is normal for you and to recognise any abnormal changes. In particular, you should be aware of any new lumps or bumps in a breast or armpit, a change in the outline or shape of a breast, dimpling, scaling or discoloration of the skin, a non-milky nipple discharge or any other changes in the nipple. Go to your doctor if you notice anything unusual or worrying.

Women aged between 50 and 70 are routinely invited for breast screening every three years. Once you reach the upper age limit for routine invitations for breast screening, you are encouraged to make your own appointment, particularly if you are taking HRT.

Keep up to date with smear tests
Cervical screening or the 'smear test' helps prevent

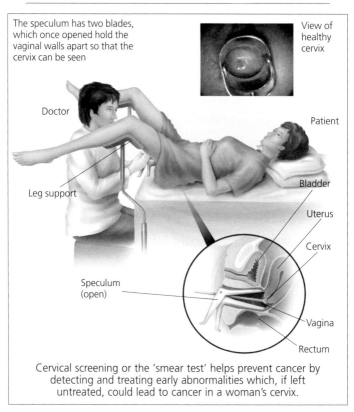

The speculum has two blades, which once opened hold the vaginal walls apart so that the cervix can be seen

View of healthy cervix

Doctor

Patient

Leg support

Bladder

Uterus

Cervix

Speculum (open)

Vagina

Rectum

Cervical screening or the 'smear test' helps prevent cancer by detecting and treating early abnormalities which, if left untreated, could lead to cancer in a woman's cervix.

cancer by detecting and treating early abnormalities which, if left untreated, could lead to cancer in a woman's cervix (the neck of the uterus). Early detection and treatment can prevent 80 to 90 per cent of cancers developing. All women between the ages of 25 and 64 are eligible for a free cervical smear test every three to five years.

If you have any tests such as a cervical smear or mammogram, ask how long it is likely to take before you will get the results. If you don't hear within a couple of weeks of this date, contact the clinic or your doctor.

Other points

See your doctor if you:

- have any unusual bleeding or very heavy or prolonged bleeding
- notice changes in your usual menstrual pattern
- have bleeding more than six months after your last period
- bleed after sexual intercourse
- notice any new breast lumps or changes in lumps that have been checked in the past
- have a discharge from your nipple(s)
- notice puckering of your breast skin, like the skin of an orange
- have any concerns or worries about your health.

KEY POINTS

- Try simple measures and lifestyle changes first
- Stop smoking and eat a healthy diet
- Maintain a healthy weight
- Take regular exercise
- Drink alcohol in moderation
- Check your breasts regularly
- Be sure to attend for routine cervical smears and breast check/mammogram appointments

Replacing the hormones (HRT)

What is HRT?

Hormone replacement therapy (HRT) does exactly what its name suggests – it replaces the ovarian hormones, estrogen and progesterone, that are no longer produced when the ovaries cease to function at the time of the menopause.

Why take HRT?

HRT is the most effective treatment for the symptoms of estrogen deficiency. The most common symptoms are hot flushes and night sweats but many women also suffer vaginal dryness and urinary frequency and urgency. Women at risk of osteoporosis benefit from HRT, although non-hormonal options are now also available.

How long has HRT been available?

Many women mistakenly believe that HRT is a new invention. In fact, written accounts exist from every era: even the ancient Egyptians sought ways to provide relief. The first documented prescription for HRT was in 1896 when a German gynaecologist gave 'ovarian therapy' to a 23-year-old woman who had had her ovaries removed.

However, early trials of HRT achieved little, because natural estrogen is poorly absorbed when taken orally. The breakthrough came in the 1930s when attempts at manufacturing synthetic estrogen were successful. At the same time, natural 'conjugated equine estrogens', a mixture of several different estrogens extracted from the urine of pregnant mares, were shown to be effective when taken by mouth. HRT was born and quickly became available commercially. Over the years, further developments have enabled natural human estrogens to be produced. Most types of HRT available in the UK now contain estrogen that is structurally indistinguishable from estrogen produced by the human ovaries.

Feminine forever?

The 1960s heralded a boom in HRT when Robert Wilson published the highly debated best-seller *Feminine Forever*. He maintained that the menopause was an estrogen deficiency disease that should be treated with estrogen to prevent the inevitable 'living decay'. This led to the myth that estrogen could be used as a panacea for all the effects of ageing.

Healing or harm?

By the mid-1970s doctors had noticed an increase in cancer of the lining of the uterus, or endometrium, in women taking estrogen. The estrogen was stimulating growth of the endometrium resulting in the formation of potentially cancerous cells. Fortunately, a simple means to protect the uterus was found – progestogen (synthetic progesterone) was combined with the estrogen. Progestogen opposes the effect of estrogen on the endometrium, preventing cancerous changes. Hence an estrogen/progestogen combination is now generally recommended for women with a uterus whereas women who have had a hysterectomy need take only estrogen.

Numerous studies followed suggesting that HRT did not just treat symptoms of the menopause, it also prevented the long-term consequences of estrogen deficiency: osteoporosis, heart attacks and strokes.

Prescription of HRT continued to rise but not everyone was so convinced of the benefits. Some doctors considered that the 'healthy user effect' explained the positive effects of HRT. The 'healthy user effect' suggested that women taking HRT might be more likely to look after themselves in other ways such as not smoking, looking after their diet and taking regular exercise. So these women would be at a lower risk of osteoporosis, heart disease and strokes, whether or not they took HRT.

More recent studies have tried to account for this and consider the overall risks versus benefits of HRT. All the trials have confirmed the benefits of HRT on osteoporosis, and have been consistent in showing an increasing risk of breast cancer associated with duration of use of combined estrogen and progestogen taken by women who have not had a hysterectomy. In contrast, there appeared to be no increased risk in breast cancer in women who had a hysterectomy and were using estrogen-only therapy.

Another finding has been the need to start HRT early postmenopause for cardiovascular benefit.

The implications of studies on HRT

Barely a month passes without another headline in the press about HRT. Notably, though, most of the headlines report possible risks rather than benefits.

Major studies reported were the Heart and Estrogen/Progestogen Replacement Study (HERS) and the Women's Health Initiative (WHI) study. Both studies were undertaken in the USA. Half the women in each study were randomly assigned to receive the hormone medication and the other half to receive inactive pills (placebo).

Neither the study participants nor the researchers knew who was taking hormones or who was taking placebo. Medical studies with this design are known as randomised, placebo-controlled, double-masked, clinical trials. They are considered to be the 'gold-standard' trial design to demonstrate a cause-and-effect connection between a particular medical condition and treatment.

In contrast, observational studies can be misleading. An example is the UK Million Women Study, which claimed that HRT nearly doubles the risk of breast cancer. These results conflict with those from placebo-controlled trials.

Heart and Estrogen/Progestogen Replacement Study

The HERS was designed to look at the effect of HRT on the rate of recurrent heart problems in women who already had heart disease. In all, 2,763 post-menopausal women, with an average age of 67, participated. None of the women had had a hysterectomy. Half of the women were given estrogen and progestogen every day; the other half took placebo. The study found that taking estrogen and progestogen for up to four years did not prevent further heart attacks or death from previous heart disease, despite there being a positive effect of HRT on cholesterol.

In the first year of the study there was an increased number of heart problems in the women taking active (HRT) medication compared with the inactive (placebo) group. However, after two or more years, the active group had fewer heart problems. This led the investigators to conclude that HRT should not be started by women in order to prevent heart problems. However, they also stated that it might be appropriate for women to continue HRT if they are already taking it when they develop a heart problem. This is because of the possible benefit from longer treatment.

Women's Health Initiative study

The WHI study is a set of clinical trials and an observational study set up by the National Institutes of Health (NIH) in the USA. It was designed to test the risks and benefits of postmenopausal hormone therapy, diet modification, and calcium and vitamin D supplements on heart disease, breast and colorectal cancer, and bone fractures in postmenopausal women. More than 160,000 women aged 50–79 were enrolled as WHI participants between 1993 and 1998.

The hormone trial had two arms: daily estrogen and progestogen given to women with a uterus and daily estrogen-only given to women who had had a hysterectomy. The trial was designed primarily to assess the benefit of hormones on the risk of heart disease, because the results of previous studies had suggested that hormones reduced this risk. At the same time, the trial assessed the risk of breast cancer, which was thought to increase with the duration of hormone use.

The estrogen/progestogen arm was expected to run until 2005 but was stopped in 2002 as a greater than anticipated number of breast cancers occurred in the women taking hormones compared with those taking placebo. The NIH felt that the potential risks of this particular type of HRT in this particular group of women outweighed the benefits. The essential findings were that, over 5.2 years of follow-up, women taking HRT had more heart attacks, strokes, blood clots and breast cancers compared with women taking placebo. However, women taking HRT had fewer bone fractures and colorectal cancers.

Similarly, the estrogen-only arm was stopped early in 2004 because the NIH believed that there were enough data to answer the main study question, and the balance of benefits and risks was not likely to change further. Like the estrogen/progestogen study, the estrogen-only study also noted in the active (HRT) group an increased number of strokes during the 6.8 years of follow-up and fewer fractures. There was a difference in the number of colorectal cancers or heart attacks between active and placebo treatment.

A follow-up to this study looked at the women taking estrogen-only HRT. Compared with women taking placebo, HRT users who had no strong family history of breast cancer were over 20 per cent less likely to develop breast cancer and over 60 per cent less likely to die from breast cancer.

What do these results mean?

It is very important to be aware that these results apply only to the specific type of HRT used, the route of delivery, the dose and the type of progestogen – in this case tablets of 0.625 mg conjugated equine estrogens taken daily with or without 2.5 mg medroxyprogesterone acetate.

Conjugated oral estrogens derived from the urine of pregnant mares may not have the same effects as human estrogens or other non-oral routes of estrogen such as skin patches or gels.

Although the type of HRT used was typical at the time these trials were designed, most HRT that we use now contains estradiol, the same estrogen produced by human ovaries. Furthermore, HRT is increasingly being prescribed at lower doses, by non-oral routes and containing different types of progestogens.

Another criticism of the WHI study is that it included women with an average age of 63 who had been exposed to estrogens for around 10 years. This is not the typical user, as most women start HRT around the age of 50 for a specific reason such as control of hot flushes or night sweats. Older women will have been deficient of estrogen for several years and will have a different response to estrogen from those who are closer to the menopause when they start to take it.

With more than 10 years since the HERS and WHO studies were published, the findings have been extensively reviewed. When data from the younger women in the WHI study are analysed, there is actually a reduced risk of heart attacks in this group. These findings have been confirmed in more recent studies of HRT given to women soon after the menopause. It has also been shown that starting HRT around the menopause helps prevent the build-up of cholesterol in the blood vessels that affect heart disease. In addition, studies show that HRT has benefits on weight, insulin levels and blood pressure.

The bottom line is that women who start HRT within 10 years of the menopause are likely to have a reduced risk of heart attacks. In contrast, women who start HRT many years beyond the menopause may have an initial increase in risk of heart attacks although, if they continue HRT, long-term use will actually reduce the risk of heart attacks. We know that there are very few risks associated with short-term use of HRT for women starting to take it around age 50 for menopausal symptoms. However, we still don't know the risks and benefits if the same women decide to continue HRT long term, that is, for more than five or ten years. Nor do we really know which is the best type of HRT to take.

In the meantime, the choice of HRT remains individual – each woman has a personal set of risks and benefits.

When reading through this book, it might be helpful to note down your own potential risks and benefits to help you consider what is right for you.

Risks and benefits of HRT

Balancing the risks (on the left of the chart) with the benefits (on the right of the chart) will depend on your individual health concerns.

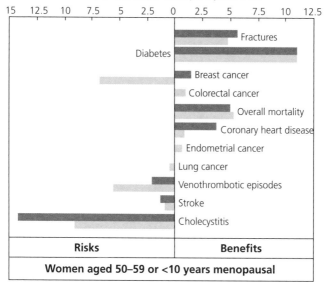

Number of women per 1,000 per 5 years of use

Risks	Benefits

Women aged 50–59 or <10 years menopausal

■ Estrogen   ▨ Estrogen + progesterone

Cholecystitis is inflammation of the gallbladder; venothrombotic episodes are blood clots in the veins; and endometrial cancer is cancer of the womb.

KEY POINTS

■ HRT aims to restore estrogen levels using natural estrogen in doses that mimic the average levels produced during the normal menstrual cycle

■ HRT is not a panacea for the effects of ageing

■ Many doctors in the UK recommend non-oral routes of estradiol, the same estrogen made naturally by the ovaries

■ There is still a great deal of research necessary to find the most effective and safest type of HRT

■ The choice of whether or not to use HRT is individual and should be based on your own balance of potential risks and benefits

■ HRT should be started as close to the menopause as possible in the lowest effective dose needed to control menopause symptoms

The benefits of HRT

Who can benefit from HRT?

HRT can benefit several groups of women. These are considered below.

Women who have an early menopause

The average age at menopause is 51, but it can occur in younger women. If you have a menopause before the age of 40, it is recognised as a premature menopause.

Often no cause for a premature menopause is found but it can also be a result of radiotherapy or chemotherapy for cancer, or following surgical removal of the ovaries (oophorectomy). Women who have a hysterectomy but retain their ovaries frequently reach menopause a few years earlier than would otherwise have occurred.

Women who have an untreated premature menopause are at particular risk of developing osteoporosis and heart disease. They are more likely to die at a younger age than women who have the menopause at the usual time.

To reduce these risks, HRT is usually recommended until at least the age of 50. Unlike HRT used beyond the average age at menopause, HRT for a premature menopause is merely replacing hormones that would normally be present. There is no evidence that HRT increases the risk of breast cancer, thrombosis or strokes over and above that found in menstruating women with a normally timed menopause. After 50, HRT can be continued if there are reasons to do so and its use should be reviewed annually.

Women with menopausal symptoms

HRT is very effective in relieving the symptoms of the menopause. The lowest dose of estrogen necessary to control symptoms is recommended. Hot flushes and night sweats usually improve within a few weeks of starting treatment. Vaginal dryness or soreness and urinary urgency and frequency may take longer to respond. Most women using HRT solely for control of menopausal symptoms should not need to take it for more than five years, although longer treatment may be necessary if symptoms recur when HRT is stopped. It is important gradually to reduce HRT over two or three months to assess the return of any symptoms. If HRT is stopped too quickly flushes and sweats will return just because of the sudden drop in hormone levels.

Women at risk of osteoporosis

Osteoporosis is a disease in which bones become more fragile and so more likely to break.

Estrogen plays an important role in building and maintaining bone. Throughout a person's life, old bone breaks down and new bone forms in the skeleton. In childhood and adolescence, new bone is formed faster

Effects of osteoporosis

Healthy bone has a resilient internal structure. Osteoporotic bone is more fragile and prone to fracture (break).

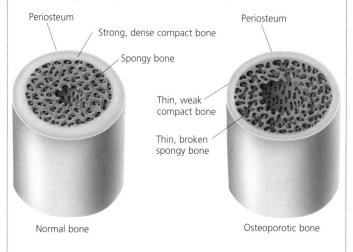

Periosteum

Strong, dense compact bone

Spongy bone

Periosteum

Thin, weak compact bone

Thin, broken spongy bone

Normal bone

Osteoporotic bone

than old bone is broken down, and the bones become larger, heavier and denser. Women usually have their peak amount of bone around age 35.

When estrogen levels fall following the menopause, the rate of bone loss increases and less new bone is formed. In some women, the bone loss can be so great that the bones become osteoporotic and the risk of fractures increases. About one in three women over the age of 50 fractures a bone as a result of osteoporosis.

HRT prevents osteoporosis but needs to be continued for life because bone strength starts to fall when treatment is stopped. Within five years of stopping HRT, the benefit of HRT on bone has been lost. This means that, unless a woman is at particular risk of osteoporosis, the risks of long-term HRT may outweigh the benefits in preventing osteoporosis.

Osteoporosis and bone fracture

Wrist and hip fractures are common symptoms of osteoporosis, causing pain and disability.

1. Hip fracture

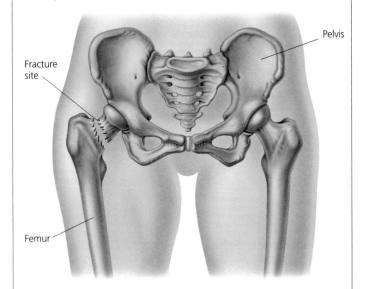

Pelvis

Fracture site

Femur

2. Wrist fracture

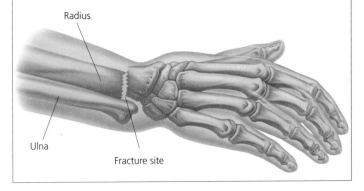

Radius

Ulna

Fracture site

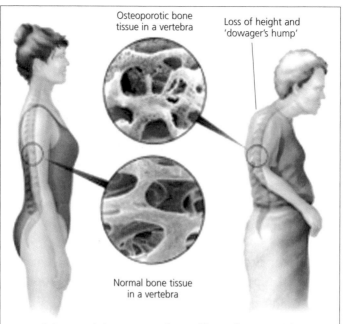

Osteoporotic bone tissue in a vertebra

Loss of height and 'dowager's hump'

Normal bone tissue in a vertebra

Osteoporosis is a common form of bone disease mainly affecting women after the menopause. Hormonal changes lead to a thinning of the interior structure of the bones, making them weaker and more prone to fracture. Weakened vertebrae may become crushed, causing loss of height and severe bending forwards, giving a hunched appearance.

How is osteoporosis diagnosed?

Osteoporosis can be confirmed by measuring bone mineral density using dual-energy X-ray absorptiometry (DXA). HRT is effective at building bone and preventing hip and vertebral fractures but, because of the balance of risks and benefits, current advice from the regulatory authorities is that HRT should not be used as a first-line treatment for osteoporosis. However, HRT may be considered for individual women with established bone loss who are unable to take alternative treatment or for whom other treatments have been unsuccessful.

Bone density measurement

The most widely used technique is using a DXA scan to produce a value for bone mineral density.

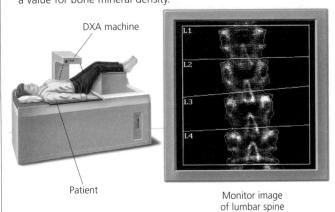

DXA machine

Patient

Monitor image
of lumbar spine

Risk factors for osteoporosis

The table on page 51 shows factors associated with increased risk of osteoporosis; the more risk factors you have, the higher your personal risk.

Increased age

The older you are, the greater your risk of fractures.

High alcohol intake

Following current recommendations, women should stick to a limit of 14 units of alcohol, ideally spread evenly over a week. One unit is equivalent to a small glass of wine, a single measure of spirits or half a pint of beer. If you keep within this limit, it is unlikely that alcohol will be detrimental to your health and may even give some protection against heart disease. Moderate-to-heavy drinking, more than three to five units a day, is associated with an increased fracture risk.

Major risk factors for osteoporosis

- Early menopause
- Increased age
- High alcohol consumption
- Smoking
- Low body mass index
- Family history
- Lack of exercise
- Extended bed rest
- Calcium-deficient diet
- History of infrequent or absent periods
- Certain medical conditions
- Lack of exposure to daylight
- Previous fractures
- Certain racial origins
- Prolonged steroid use

Factors protective for osteoporosis

- Oral contraception use
- High number of pregnancies

Smoking
Chemicals from tobacco smoke in the bloodstream can affect bones and hasten bone loss.

Low body mass index
How to calculate your body mass index (BMI) is explained in 'Helping yourself' (on page 30). The ideal BMI is between 18.5 and 24.9. A BMI of less than 18.5 is associated with an increased risk of osteoporosis and fractures. A BMI of over 25 indicates an increased risk of high blood pressure, diabetes and heart disease.

Family history
If a blood relative, particularly your mother, has lost height or has fractured a hip or wrist through

osteoporosis, it is more likely that you will also fracture a bone.

Lack of exercise

Exercise helps strengthen bones, so if you drive to a sedentary job you are at greater risk of osteoporosis than someone who is on her feet all day. Regular weight-bearing exercise is best for bones, such as brisk walking, aerobics or dancing.

Other risk factors
Extended rest

Bed rest leads to rapid bone loss. If it is necessary to stay in bed for extended periods of time, physiotherapy and simple exercise will help reduce bone loss.

High caffeine intake

Drinking copious cups of coffee or strong tea during the day has been linked to osteoporosis. It is difficult to state a maximum level of intake, although no more than two to four cups a day is generally recommended. Watch for caffeine in other products, particularly canned colas and some health drinks.

Calcium-deficient diet

Adequate amounts of calcium are essential to maintain bone strength. Women need at least 700 to 1,200 mg a day. If you restrict calcium-rich dairy products in your diet, it may be worth boosting your calcium with a supplement.

History of infrequent or absent periods

Amenorrhoea (lack of menstrual periods) for longer than one year is associated with insufficient estrogen to maintain a normal menstrual cycle. Estrogen deficiency is the result. Long periods of dieting and anorexia nervosa are common causes in young women. Young gymnasts or marathon runners are also at risk. Some treatments for endometriosis (when the uterine lining is found in tissues outside the uterus) stimulate a temporary menopause by switching off the production of estrogen. All these situations can increase the risk of estrogen deficiency symptoms and diseases.

Certain medical conditions

An overactive thyroid increases the resting metabolic rate, speeding up the normal process of bone formation and breakdown, which can lead to osteoporosis. Other medical conditions associated with an increased risk of osteoporosis include Cushing's disease, inflammatory bowel disease, chronic liver disease, coeliac disease and rheumatoid arthritis.

Lack of daylight

Elderly women often stay indoors and get little sunlight on their skin. In certain cultures women are heavily covered in dark clothing and, particularly if they live in Europe, minimal daylight reaches their skin. Sunlight is very important because it stimulates the production of vitamin D in the skin. Vitamin D aids the absorption of calcium from food, helping bones to stay strong and healthy. Only 10 to 15 minutes of sun exposure at least twice a week to the face, arms, hands or back, without sunscreen, is usually sufficient to provide adequate vitamin D.

Previous fractures

Previous fractures suggest existing osteoporosis, increasing the likelihood of further broken bones.

Certain racial origins

Women of African–Caribbean racial origin achieve a 10 per cent greater peak bone mass than women of European extraction, hence women of European racial origin are at greater risk of osteoporosis.

Prolonged steroid use

Prolonged use of oral steroids, over five milligrams each day for more than three months, is linked to osteoporosis. Steroids are usually prescribed for conditions such as severe asthma or other autoimmune diseases. In these conditions the body's protective mechanisms are disrupted and normal tissue is seen as a foreign body that should be destroyed.

Short-term courses of steroids, taken for one or two weeks, are not associated with increased risks unless repeated frequently. If you are on long-term steroid therapy, speak to your doctor to discuss alternative therapy and ways that you can prevent osteoporosis developing.

Protective factors
Oral contraceptive use

Studies have shown a lower risk of fractures in women who have taken combined oral contraceptives for five years or more during their 30s or 40s (see page 130).

High number of pregnancies

Research shows an increase in bone density with increasing parity (the number of pregnancies a woman delivers past 28 weeks). The positive effect on bone density has been seen in both pre- and post-menopausal women. One study concluded that women with three or more children had a 30–40 per cent reduction in hip fracture risk when compared with nulliparous women (those who have never given birth).

Osteoporosis: the alternatives to HRT

For a fuller explanation of these treatments see the Family Doctor book *Understanding Osteoporosis*.

Bisphosphonates

Bisphosphonates are a group of medicines that include alendronate (brand or proprietary name Fosamax), etidronate (proprietary name Didronel), ibandronate (proprietary name Bonviva), risedronate (proprietary name Actonel), sodium clodronate (proprietary names Bonefos and Loron) and tiludronic acid (proprietary name Skelid), which are available on prescription. Etidronate is available in combination with calcium (proprietary name Didronel PMO). Alendronate is also available in combination with vitamin D_3 (proprietary name Fosavance).

Bisphosphonates are the most commonly used medicines to treat osteoporosis and prevent bone loss. They are the preferred choice for women in their 60s who need treatment. Long-term safety over 20 years is not known and some research suggests that, although they may increase the amount of bone, the new bone formed is not as strong as bone formed by estrogens. Bisphosphonates increase the risk of osteonecrosis of the jaw. In this condition the blood supply to the jaw bone is reduced and, without an adequate blood supply, the bone tissue dies. This is far more likely to occur in people taking bisphosphonates who also have cancer, smoke or have dental disease. To reduce the risk, make sure that you look after your teeth and visit the dentist for routine check-ups. As a result of these

Calcium supplements

Calcium supplement	Dose (milligrams)	Formulation
Adcal	600	Chewable tablets
Cacit	500	Effervescent tablets
Calcichew	500	Chewable tablets
Calcium-500	500	Tablet
Calcium gluconate	53	Tablet
Calcium lactate	39	Tablet
Calcium-Sandoz	108	Syrup
Sandocal 1000	1,000	Effervescent tablets

Amounts of calcium are shown per tablet or dose.

Combined calcium and vitamin D preparations

Preparation	Vitamin D (IU/dose)	Calcium (mg/dose)	Formulation
Adcal-D_3	400	600	Tablet
Calcium and ergocalciferol	400	97	Tablet
Calceos	400	500	Chewable tablet
Calfovit D_3	800	1,200	Powder
Kalcipos-D	800	500	Chewable tablet
Natecal D_3	400	600	Chewable tablet

Drugs for osteoporosis

Calcitonin
Miacalcic (Novartis)
- calcitonin 200 IU per spray (nasal spray)

Vitamin D
Desunin (Meda Pharmaceuticals Ltd)
- cholecalciferol 800 IU (tablets)
Fultium-D$_3$ (Internis Pharmaceuticals Ltd)
- cholecalciferol 800 IU (tablets)
Rocaltrol (Roche)
- calcitriol 0.25 µg (capsules)
- calcitriol 0.5 µg (capsules)

Bisphosphonate/vitamin D$_3$
Fosovance (MSD)
- alendronate sodium (= 70 mg alendronic acid) + 2,800 IU vitamin D$_3$ (tablets)

Bisphosphonate/calcium/vitamin D$_3$
Actonel Combi ((Warner Chilcott UK Ltd)
- risedronate sodium 35 mg (tablets)
- calcium carbonate 2,500 mg (calcium 1 g) + 880 IU vitamin D$_3$
(effervescent sachets)

Bisphosphonate
Aclasta (Novartis)
- zoledronate 5 mg (intravenous infusion) once yearly
Actonel Once a Week (Warner Chilcott UK Ltd)
- risedronate sodium 35 mg (tablets) once weekly
Bonefos (Bayer plc)
- sodium clodronate 400 mg (capsules) or 800 mg (tablets)
Bonviva (Roche)
- ibandronic acid 150 mg (tablets) once monthly
Clasteon (Beacon)
- sodium clodronate 400 mg (capsules)
Didronel (Warner Chilcott UK Ltd)
- etidronate disodium 200 mg (tablets)
Fosamax Once Weekly (MSD)
- alendronate sodium (= 70 mg alendronic acid) (tablets) once weekly
Loron (Intrapharm)
- sodium clodronate 520 mg (tablets)

Denosumab
Prolia (Amgen Ltd)
- denosumab 60 mg (subcutaneous injection) every six months

Nandrolone
Deca-Durabolin (MSD)
- nandrolone decanoate 50 mg (intramuscular injection) every three weeks

Parathyroid hormone
Preotact (Nycomed UK Ltd)
- parathyroid hormone 100 µg (subcutaneous injection)

Raloxifene
Evista (Lilly Eli)
- raloxifene 60 mg (tablets)

Strontium
Protelos (Servier)
- strontium ranelate 2 g (granules)

Teriparatide
Forsteo (Lilly Eli)
- teriparatide 20 µg (subcutaneous injection)

concerns, many specialists recommend that women who have a premature menopause and are at risk of osteoporosis would gain most benefit from HRT.

Other drugs
Other drugs available on prescription include calcitonin (Miacalcic), raloxifene (Evista), teriparatide (Forsteo) and strontium ranelate (Protelos).

Calcitonin is a hormone that slows down bone loss and increases the density of the spinal bone. However, the effects of calcitonin on fracture risk remain unclear. Raloxifene belongs to a relatively new group of drugs known as selective estrogen receptor modulators, or SERMs. These drugs are not estrogens but have estrogen-like effects on bone, increasing bone mass and reducing the risk of spinal fractures.

Teriparatide (Forsteo), a drug identical to human parathyroid hormone, is occasionally used but has to be given by daily injection under the skin of the thigh or abdomen. Unlike the bisphosphonates, teriparatide stimulates bone formation rather than just slowing down the rate at which bone is lost.

Strontium ranelate also increases bone formation as well as preventing bone loss. It is taken once daily at bedtime, dissolved in water.

Other benefits of HRT
Arthritis
Increasing evidence suggests that HRT reduces the symptoms of arthritis, although it is not licensed (see Glossary, page 18) for this indication. This is true for both osteoarthritis and rheumatoid arthritis. Although HRT does not reverse the process of these conditions,

it is a useful adjunct to conventional therapy and is worth discussing with your GP or specialist.

Colorectal cancer

The incidence of colorectal cancer is rising. Between 1971 and 1997 in the UK the total number of cases increased by 42 per cent, from 20,400 to 28,900. In 2006, over 37,000 people in the UK were diagnosed with this condition. This makes colorectal cancer the second most common cancer that affects women (after breast cancer). Recent studies suggest that HRT may reduce the risk of developing colorectal cancer by about one-third.

KEY POINTS

■ HRT is of particular benefit to women who have a premature menopause as these women are at high risk of osteoporosis in later life

■ For women who have had a premature menopause, if HRT is taken until 51 – the average age at menopause – there is no evidence of increased risks associated with its use

■ HRT is the most effective treatment for menopausal symptoms

■ HRT is one of several treatments that are effective for osteoporosis

■ HRT has been shown to reduce the risk of colorectal cancer and to improve symptoms of arthritis

■ HRT improves other estrogen-related complaints, such as joint and muscle pain, mood swings, sleep disturbances and sexual dysfunction (including libido)

The risks of HRT

What are the risks of HRT?

Although HRT can offer many benefits, for some women it can carry unacceptable potential risks. When deciding whether or not HRT is right for you, you must consider the balance between risks and benefits.

The main potential risks that have been identified are:

- breast cancer

- blood clots in the veins (venous thrombosis)

- blood clots in the arteries (heart attacks and strokes)

- cancer of the lining of the uterus (endometrium), though this can be prevented by the addition of progestogen

- ovarian cancer.

It is important to understand these risks and put them into perspective – most women taking HRT do not experience any of these problems as a direct result of taking the hormones. Furthermore, other risk factors are often more important than HRT – particularly smoking or being very overweight – in creating these problems.

Breast cancer

Women starting HRT before the age of 50 for a premature menopause do not, as we presently understand it, have an increased risk of breast cancer. This indicates that it is the duration of lifetime exposure to estrogen that is the relevant factor.

So those women who have a late natural menopause or take HRT beyond the age of 50 are at higher risk of developing breast cancer than women who have a menopause at the more usual time (51) because they will have had a greater lifetime exposure to estrogen. After stopping HRT the risk of breast cancer gradually returns to the same level as for women who have never taken HRT. By five years after stopping HRT, there is no difference in risk between women who have taken and women who have never taken HRT.

Breast cancer is not uncommon in women in later life even when not using HRT – a 50-year-old woman has a 6.1 per cent risk (61 in 1,000) of developing breast cancer over the next 30 years with no HRT.

Studies show that the type of HRT started after the menopause affects the risk of breast cancer. Estrogen-only HRT must be taken for at least five years before the risk of breast cancer increases. If taken for less than five years, it has little risk and may even reduce the risk of breast cancer. Combined estrogen/progestogen HRT, necessary for women who have not had a hysterectomy, seems to increase the risk of breast cancer. This risk begins within three to five years of starting treatment, and the risk increases with continued use.

However, it is important to put the risks associated with HRT into perspective and compare them with other risk factors. Being overweight or drinking more than 14 units of alcohol a week are stronger risk factors for breast cancer than using HRT. One study estimated that more than six per cent of breast cancers in women in the UK in 2010 were linked to alcohol consumption and nine per cent were linked to excess body weight. The same study estimated that three per cent of breast cancers were linked to HRT use.

Survival for breast cancer is much higher than in the past. Some if this is due to faster diagnosis and over a third are detected during routine breast screening. Treatment for breast cancer is also much more effective than before. Although 10-year survival rates for women diagnosed with breast cancer during 1971–5 were only 40 per cent, the rates have now doubled so that almost 80 per cent of women diagnosed with breast cancer can expect to still be alive 10 years later.

The findings highlight several important points:

- A woman's chances of developing breast cancer depend on a number of risk factors
- The extra risk from HRT is small.

Different types of HRT

Most women are now given different types of HRT to those used in the studies and we do not know whether or not the findings can be extended to these newer types of HRT. Since then natural estradiol has become available and is most commonly used.

Different ways of taking HRT

An increasing number of women use non-oral HRT such as patches and gels, which enables a smaller dose of HRT to be given with the same effect as a higher dose of tablets. This is because, when a tablet is swallowed, the hormones are absorbed in the gut and have to pass through the liver before they reach the bloodstream. Once in the bloodstream, the hormones can be circulated all around the body. However, the liver breaks down hormones, so not all the dose of hormones swallowed actually reaches the blood. In contrast, patches and gels enable hormones to pass through the skin, directly into the bloodstream.

In the light of these results, however, women who haven't had a hysterectomy may be tempted to take estrogen-only HRT, but it must be remembered that progestogen is necessary to protect against endometrial cancer (see page 120).

Early onset of menstruation

The risk of developing breast cancer appears to be related to the number of years of exposure to estrogen and progestogen. Early onset of menstruation before the age of 12 years is associated with about a twofold increase in the risk of breast cancer.

Premature menopause

Women who have premature menopause will have a reduction in the risk of developing breast cancer. These women typically may have a 50 per cent reduction in the risk of breast cancer, but are at much higher risk for heart disease and osteoporosis.

Pregnancy

Never having given birth to a child and late age at first birth both increase the lifetime incidence of breast cancer. The highest risk women are those who have a first child after the age of 35; these women appear to be at even higher risk than women who have never had a full-term pregnancy.

Breast-feeding

The role of the protective effect of breast-feeding on breast cancer is not very clear, but there is some evidence to suggest that this may be the case.

Body weight

A high body mass index (BMI), over 30, also increases the risk of breast cancer by 50 per cent compared with women with a normal BMI of 25 or lower.

Family history

Current medical research suggests that there may be an

Non-HRT risk factors for breast cancer

- Family history
- Older age at birth of first child
- Late menopause
- Early menarche (age at first period)
- Postmenopausal obesity
- Alcohol – more than two to three units/day

inherited risk of breast cancer. A family history of breast cancer in a close relative usually indicates a greater personal risk but there is no evidence to show that using HRT further increases the risk. However, if you are at high risk of breast cancer and have a low risk of osteoporosis and minimal menopausal symptoms, there is little advantage in taking HRT. If you are experiencing marked flushes and sweats, and have no risk factors for breast cancer, HRT might be a good choice for you.

HRT for women treated for breast cancer

Although HRT is increasingly considered to be an effective option for severe flushes and sweats resulting from the treatment of breast cancer, its use is controversial and the results of studies are conflicting. However, HRT is offered in several specialist breast cancer centres where the doctors have more experience of using HRT in these circumstances. Alternative approaches to debilitating menopausal symptoms in women treated for breast cancer include vaginal estrogen (creams, pessaries, tablets and rings) to help vaginal dryness. For hot flushes and sweats, non-hormonal treatments such as selective serotonin reuptake inhibitors (SSRIs – antidepressants) may help (see page 126).

Venous thrombosis

Increasing age is the main risk for venous thrombosis (blood clots in veins). However, research suggests that women using HRT are more likely to develop venous thrombosis than women of a similar age who are not using HRT, especially in the first year of use. About 3 per 1,000 women in their 50s who do not use HRT are likely to have a venous thrombosis in any 5-year period compared with 7 per 1,000 women of the same age

Venous thrombosis

Deep vein thrombosis is a condition in which a blood clot forms in a large vein, usually in the leg. There is a risk that the clot may travel through the heart and become lodged in another part of the body, for instance a blood vessel supplying the lungs, which can be fatal.

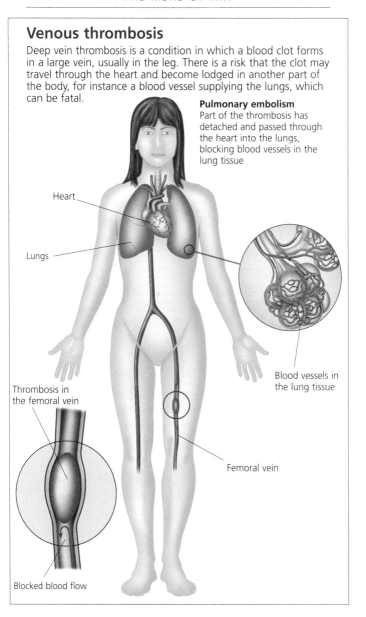

Pulmonary embolism
Part of the thrombosis has detached and passed through the heart into the lungs, blocking blood vessels in the lung tissue

Heart

Lungs

Blood vessels in the lung tissue

Thrombosis in the femoral vein

Femoral vein

Blocked blood flow

Non-HRT risk factors for venous thrombosis

- Severe varicose veins
- Obesity
- Increased age
- Inactivity
- Diabetes
- High blood pressure

who take HRT.

By the time they reach their 60s, the risk in non-users increases to 8 per 1,000 women in a 5-year period compared with 17 per 1,000 women taking HRT. However, published data suggest that non-oral HRT such as patches and gels is less likely to increase the risk of venous thrombosis than HRT tablets.

If you have multiple risk factors for venous thrombosis (see above), HRT is probably best avoided. If you have major surgery and will be off your feet for a while, you will probably be given drugs to help prevent blood clots. Some doctors advise stopping HRT four to six weeks before major surgery. You can usually start HRT again once you are fully mobile.

If you or a close relative has had an unexplained venous thrombosis under the age of 45, you may need to have a blood test to check your blood clotting before you can take HRT. This can identify those women who have a genetic risk factor for venous thrombosis, the most common of which is known as factor V Leiden. This genetic condition affects around five per cent of the population and causes an increased tendency for blood to clot. People carrying the factor V Leiden gene have a five times greater risk of developing a blood clot than the rest of the population.

Heart attacks and strokes

It is quite rare for a woman to suffer a heart attack or a stroke before the menopause; the incidence starts to rise in postmenopausal women. Heart disease is now recognised as the leading cause of early death in women, more significant than any type of cancer. Twenty per cent of postmenopausal women are at risk of stroke, with an eight per cent chance of death. Likewise, postmenopausal women have a 46 per cent chance of developing coronary heart disease at some point with a one in three chance of it causing death.

With respect to stroke, about 3 out of 1,000 women in their 50s not using HRT can expect to have a stroke in any 5-year period. For women of a similar age who use HRT for 5 years, the figure rises to 4 per 1,000. The risk rises with age, so the risk in non-HRT users in their 60s is 11 per 1,000 in any 5-year period compared with 15 per 1,000 women of the same age using HRT.

Until recently, it was always thought that HRT protected against heart disease and strokes. This was based on observational studies, comparing HRT users with non-users. The WHI study compared postmenopausal women taking conjugated estrogen and medroxyprogesterone acetate against women taking inactive treatment. The results suggested that the risk of heart disease was increased in the first two years of use. However, the average age of women starting HRT in the study was 63 – much older than women in the observational studies, most of which looked at women starting HRT around the age of 50. The WHI study further showed that, when HRT was continued, there was a trend to reduced risk of heart disease, that is, continuing HRT reduced the risk of heart disease.

Stroke

The most common cause of a stroke is a thrombosis – when a blood vessel supplying the brain becomes blocked with a blood clot. The second most common cause of a stroke is a brain haemorrhage, of which there are two types; both involve a blood vessel bursting inside the head.

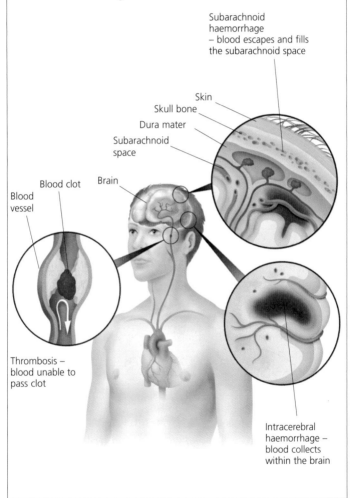

Subarachnoid haemorrhage – blood escapes and fills the subarachnoid space

Skin

Skull bone

Dura mater

Subarachnoid space

Brain

Blood clot

Blood vessel

Thrombosis – blood unable to pass clot

Intracerebral haemorrhage – blood collects within the brain

Heart disease – the process of atherosclerosis

Atherosclerosis, atheroma and hardening of the arteries are all the same thing – the process leading to the blockage or weakening of arteries.

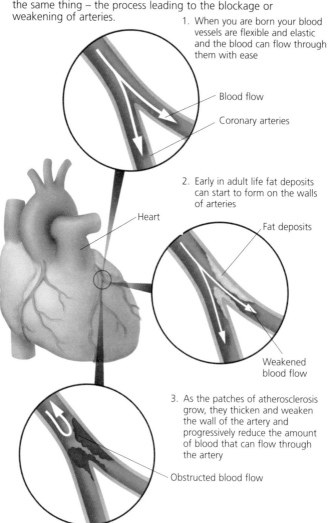

1. When you are born your blood vessels are flexible and elastic and the blood can flow through them with ease

Blood flow

Coronary arteries

Heart

2. Early in adult life fat deposits can start to form on the walls of arteries

Fat deposits

Weakened blood flow

3. As the patches of atherosclerosis grow, they thicken and weaken the wall of the artery and progressively reduce the amount of blood that can flow through the artery

Obstructed blood flow

Non-HRT risk factors for heart disease

- High blood pressure
- High cholesterol
- Smoking
- Previous heart attack or stroke
- Irregular heart beat (atrial fibrillation)
- Diabetes
- Obesity
- Personality – people who are competitive and easily stressed are more likely to develop heart disease than people who are laid back about life

Furthermore, when the age of women in the WHI study was considered, the women who were between 50 and 59 when they started the study actually had an overall reduction in the risk of heart disease. These findings could be explained by the fact that estrogen increases blood clotting, increasing the risk of stroke and heart attacks but, in the long term, can prevent a build-up of atherosclerosis in the blood vessels, reducing the risk of stroke and heart attacks.

If HRT is started in women who are used to having estrogen in the body, as are women starting HRT around the age of 50, they will be less susceptible to the clotting effects of estrogen and more likely to benefit from the long-term effects to protect against atherosclerosis. Older women starting HRT after years of estrogen deficiency will already have developed atherosclerosis and may be more susceptible to the effect of estrogen on blood clotting.

There are no data yet for other types of HRT which

may have a different effect. What is needed is a study of different types of HRT started by women aged between 45 and 56. However, until such studies are undertaken, HRT should not be started to prevent further heart attacks in women who have already had a heart attack.

If you have had angina, a heart attack or stroke in the past, you should see your doctor to discuss the possible benefits and risks of HRT for you. However, if you are already taking HRT when you have your first heart attack or stroke, there is probably no reason to stop HRT because continuing treatment may reduce your long-term risk of a repeat event.

Cancer of the uterus

Around 8 per 100,000 women a year over age 50 who are not using HRT develop cancer of the lining of the uterus (endometrial cancer). Women taking 'unopposed' estrogen-only HRT for five years have a sixfold increased risk. A breakthrough in research showed that 'opposing' the estrogen by adding progestogen reduced this risk. With combined estrogen/ progestogen HRT, the risk of endometrial cancer is at least the same as for non-HRT users, if not lower.

Ovarian cancer

There appears to be a small increase in the risk of ovarian cancer in women using HRT compared with non-users. In non-users, you would expect 2.2 women out of 1,000 to develop ovarian cancer over a 5-year period. In HRT users, this rises to 2.6 women per 1,000 over a 5-year period. This suggests that one extra woman out of 2,500 women using HRT over 5 years will develop ovarian cancer compared with a similar group of women not taking HRT.

KEY POINTS

- The potential risks of HRT use include breast and endometrial cancer, venous thrombosis and stroke

- Use of conjugated equine estrogens alone does not appear to be associated with an increased risk of breast cancer

- HRT containing conjugated equine estrogens combined with medroxyprogesterone acetate is associated with an increased risk of breast cancer

- The risk of breast cancer declines after stopping HRT and, by five years, is the same as if you have never taken it

- Taking HRT increases your risk of venous thrombosis, especially in the first year of use

- HRT started at the time of the menopause may reduce the long-term risk of heart disease

- The potential risks associated with HRT use are smaller than the health risks associated with smoking or being very overweight

Different types of HRT

Availability of HRT

Hormone replacement therapy (HRT) is available only on prescription. There are numerous different brands of HRT marketed, some containing both estrogen and progestogen, some containing estrogen only, in a variety of preparations.

Estrogen preparations

Estrogens used in HRT are either natural or synthetic. Both produce effects similar to the estrogens produced by the ovaries. Natural estrogens are similar in chemical structure to the estrogens produced by the ovaries whereas synthetic ones have a different structure. Estradiol, estrone and estriol are natural human ovarian estrogens. Equilin and 17-alpha-dihydroequilin are natural equine estrogens derived from the urine of pregnant mares. Dienoestrol, ethinylestradiol and mestranol are synthetic estrogens.

Natural estrogens, both human and equine, are preferred for HRT because they have fewer side effects. Synthetic estrogens are more potent and so are

The different types of estrogen and progestogen preparations

Although tablets are the most common form in which estrogen and progestogen preparations are supplied, HRT also comes in a variety of other forms. Systemic hormones circulate throughout the body, whereas local vaginal estrogens treat only vaginal symptoms.

Estrogen

Systemic
- Tablets
- Patches
- Gels
- Vaginal ring

Vaginal (local)
- Creams
- Pessary
- Ring
- Tablet

Progestogen

Systemic
- Tablets/Caplets
- Patches (combined with estrogen)

Intrauterine
- Levonorgestrel intrauterine system (IUS)

favoured for contraception because they suppress ovulation effectively. Estrogens are available for HRT in various forms. For systemic absorption, which means circulating in the bloodstream to all the tissues in the body, they come as tablets, patches, implants and gels, and in a vaginal ring. To apply just to your vagina (local vaginal application) you can get creams, pessaries, tablets and a vaginal ring.

Progestogen preparations

Progesterone is also produced by the ovaries, and has a very sedative effect (makes you sleepy). It is available on prescription as a tablet.

Most HRTs contain synthetic forms of progesterone called progestogens. These have similar effects to natural progesterone but are available as oral tablets that can be taken once a day or combined with estrogen in patches. Estrogen combined with cyclical progestogen is the HRT most women use if they start HRT before, or shortly after, the menopause. Estrogen is taken continuously, without a break. A monthly course of progestogen lasting 10 to 14 days mimics the natural hormone cycle in which progesterone is produced for the last 14 days of the cycle, following ovulation. As in the natural menstrual cycle, when the course of progesterone or progestogen is stopped, 'withdrawal' of the hormone results in menstrual bleeding, or a 'period'.

Most women who have gone through the menopause do not wish to return to monthly periods. To avoid this, a combination of estrogen and progestogen is taken daily. Taking both hormones together prevents any thickening of the uterine lining, making a withdrawal bleed unnecessary while providing protection against endometrial cancer.

Oral tablets
Estrogen

HRT is most commonly prescribed as tablets. If you have had a hysterectomy, only estrogen treatment is necessary, because you do not need to take progestogen with the estrogen to protect your uterus.

You should take the tablets every day, without a break, at about the same time each day.

Progestogen

If your periods have not stopped and you have not had a hysterectomy, you need to take a course of progestogen every month, for about 10 to 14 days, in order to mimic the natural menstrual cycle. This is usually available in calendar packs, the progestogen combined with estrogen, so that you do not have to work out when to take them. From around the age of 55 when most women have completely stopped their periods, it is possible to take progestogens together with estrogen every day – a period-free preparation.

For women who want to take progestogen with their own choice of estrogen, they are also available separately. If used this way, many doctors recommend that women take the progestogen for the first 10 to 14 days of every calendar month, for instance starting 1 March, 1 April and so on. This has the advantage that the type and dose of estrogen and progestogen can be adjusted more easily than standard packs. A withdrawal bleed or period should start around the middle of each month, which makes it easy for the doctor to assess if there is any irregular bleeding that may need further investigation.

Women whose last natural period was more than one year ago can take the same dose of progestogen continuously every day.

Advantages of tablets

Most people find tablets easy to take and their effects are quickly reversed if they decide to discontinue treatment (see page 105 for section on stopping HRT).

Disadvantages of tablets

It is not always easy to remember to take tablets every day, and even more difficult to remember when people are away from home. Missing a tablet can trigger fluctuations in hormone levels and irregular bleeding.

It is necessary to take much higher doses of hormones by mouth to allow for huge losses because the hormones are absorbed from the gut and pass through the liver where they are usually broken down and excreted from the body. Such doses can increase side effects. Nausea is more common with tablets than with other routes but can be minimised by taking the tablet with food or at bedtime. Rarely, oral estrogen is so poorly absorbed that menopausal symptoms are not controlled and an alternative route of HRT administration is recommended.

Skin patches
Estrogen

Skin patches provide a means of delivering the hormones directly to the bloodstream through the skin, bypassing the liver. Patches are applied once or twice weekly, depending on the brand. The 'matrix' patches, which look just like a thin sheet of plastic, are generally well tolerated.

To use patches, remove the backing sheet and stick onto clean, dry skin, free from talcum powder, bath oils or body cream. The best site is the upper buttock. Press the patch firmly on your skin for about 10 seconds, then run your fingers around the edges to seal it.

You can keep the patch on when you have a bath or go swimming, although it can be removed temporarily for half an hour or so if you prefer – keep the backing sheet to stick the patch on to until you need it again. Cover the patch when sunbathing and remove it if you are using a sunbed to avoid the sun irritating the skin around the patch. When replacing patches, change the site, for example alternate buttocks, so that you are not sticking the patch in the same place each time as the skin can become red and sore underneath it.

Estrogen/progestogen combinations

Patches are available that produce a monthly bleed. As with the tablets, they are packaged so that ones containing both estrogen and progestogen are used for the first two weeks and estrogen-only patches for the second two weeks.

Postmenopausal women who do not want periods can use combined estrogen/progestogen patches continuously.

Advantages of patches

Unlike tablets, hormones from patches do not pass through the stomach and liver first, so the dose can be lower, reducing side effects. The hormone levels are also much more constant with patches than with tablets. There are several different strengths available.

Disadvantages of patches

The main disadvantage is that there are not yet many varieties available. At present there is only one dose strength of a combined patch with no choice of the type of estrogen and progestogen, so adjusting the dose can be difficult.

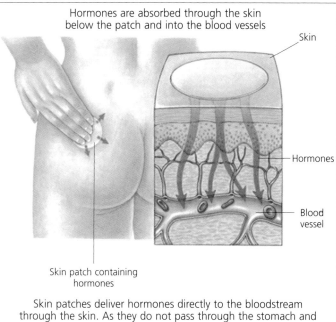

Hormones are absorbed through the skin below the patch and into the blood vessels

Skin

Hormones

Blood vessel

Skin patch containing hormones

Skin patches deliver hormones directly to the bloodstream through the skin. As they do not pass through the stomach and liver first, as tablets do, the required dose is much lower, thus reducing the side effects.

Occasionally, patches do not stick very well, particularly in hot, sticky weather, but this can easily be remedied by covering the patch with two-inch surgical tape.

Even if a different site is used each time as recommended, it is normal for the skin underneath the patch to redden. However, a few women develop a severe skin reaction that prohibits further use. Switching to a different brand of patch can occasionally help.

Gel

Estrogen and testosterone, but not progestogen, are available as a gel. The gel is applied daily to the arms and shoulders, or thighs, and absorbed through the skin into the bloodstream.

Advantages of gel
Many women find a gel convenient and easy to use, with few side effects. Unlike some estrogen patches, skin irritation is rarely a problem. The dose is easy to change and balance against symptoms.

Disadvantages of gel
Some women worry that they are not applying the gel to the correct amount of skin. On a practical note, it is easiest just to apply the gel to the upper thighs, like a skin cream, without worrying too much about how much skin is covered. The gel dries quickly and it is only necessary to wait five minutes at most before dressing. Avoid using other skin products or washing the area for an hour after application. Unless the woman has had a hysterectomy, additional progestogen is necessary.

Implants
Estrogen
In the UK, estrogen implants are currently only available in specialist clinics that import them from the USA. Availability of testosterone implants is also limited. Small pellets of estrogen, inserted into the fat under the skin of the lower abdomen or buttock, typically last for about six months. The downside is that, if the woman decides to stop HRT, they cannot easily be removed. Insertion is a simple procedure that can be done at the local surgery or in the hospital outpatient department. An injection of a local anaesthetic is given to numb the skin before a small cut is made. After the implant is inserted, the wound is

closed with a stitch or small strips of sticky tape (Steri-Strips).

Testosterone

Testosterone is the main male hormone, although the ovaries produce small amounts. The precise role of testosterone in women is unclear, although there is evidence that low testosterone levels can adversely affect mood, energy and libido. Although adequate estrogen replacement often resolves these symptoms, testosterone is sometimes recommended for women with loss of sexual desire, particularly if they have had their ovaries removed and cannot produce testosterone themselves. Testosterone is not licensed for women in the UK but can be prescribed 'off-licence'.

Advantages of implants

The advantage of implants is that, once inserted, you can forget about HRT for at least six months. The implants dissolve slowly and provide constant levels of hormone. Implants produce the highest levels of estrogen of all forms of HRT, with greatest effect on bone density.

Disadvantages of implants

Minor surgery is needed every six months. Although the pellets usually dissolve completely within about six months, you are often left with small lumps of fibrous tissue under the skin. You will also have small scars where the implants were inserted. The main disadvantage is that, if this method does not suit you, it is virtually impossible to remove the pellet once implanted.

An occasional problem is that the implants last increasingly shorter periods of time after each insertion,

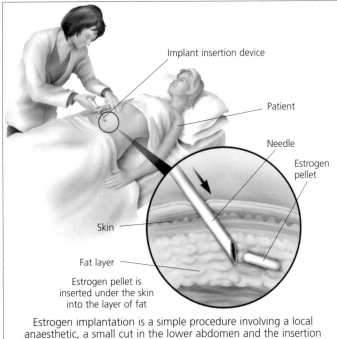

Estrogen implantation is a simple procedure involving a local anaesthetic, a small cut in the lower abdomen and the insertion of an estrogen pellet into the layer of fat under the skin. The wound is then closed with a stitch or a piece of tape.

so that menopausal symptoms return only two or three months after the last implant. Paradoxically, if estrogen levels are measured, they are very high and it seems as if these women have developed some immunity to the effects of the implant. This phenomenon is known as 'tachyphylaxis' and seems to occur only with implants. Unfortunately, the only way to treat this is to withhold further implants until the estrogen levels fall to within the normal range. Tachyphylaxis can usually be avoided by measuring estrogen levels before each implant is inserted to ensure that no more than the necessary dose is given. Many doctors will not insert a new implant without knowing the estrogen levels at the time of insertion.

Implants are rarely used in women who have not had a hysterectomy because the sustained effect of estrogen on the endometrium means that it is imperative that progestogen is taken regularly until the estrogen is completely used up. This may be up to a couple of years after the final implant. This can be a problem for women who experience unwanted side effects of progestogen.

Vaginal (local) estrogen

Vaginal creams and pessaries are useful for women who have mostly vaginal symptoms. They are simple and easy to use but can be a bit messy. Vaginal tablets are a more convenient option. All are placed directly into the vagina.

Advantages of local estrogen

Used correctly there is little risk associated with them. They are extremely useful for women with few symptoms other than a dry vagina or bladder problems. They can be used in addition to standard HRT regimens if vaginal dryness is a continuing problem, although a check with a doctor must be made to exclude non-hormonal causes.

Disadvantages of local estrogen

Creams and pessaries can be messy. Estrogen tablets, which come with an applicator ensuring that the estrogen is placed high in the vagina, and a vaginal ring, are alternative options.

Use them strictly as prescribed because some types of local estrogen don't just act locally but are absorbed into the bloodstream. In this case, unless the woman has had a hysterectomy, it may be necessary to take additional progestogen. A doctor can advise about the need for this.

Other forms of progestogen
Natural progesterone
Natural progesterone, structurally the same as progesterone from the ovaries, is available as Utrogestan. It is generally used every other day for 12 days of the cycle to stimulate a withdrawal bleed. In some clinical trials it has been used twice weekly together with estrogen as part of a continuous combined regimen.

Rectal or vaginal suppositories of natural progesterone are sometimes used for women experiencing bad side effects from progestogen, but doctors rarely prescribe these because they are not licensed (see Glossary, page 148) for HRT.

Natural progesterone creams can be purchased from health-food shops. Used alone, these can alleviate some menopausal symptoms. However, they should not be used as the progestogen component of combined HRT because they do not provide adequate endometrial protection.

Levonorgestrel intrauterine system
The levonorgestrel **i**ntra**u**terine **s**ystem, or IUS (proprietary name Mirena), is a highly effective contraceptive. It has a reservoir of the progestogen levonorgestrel, which is slowly released directly into the uterus, keeping the lining of the uterus thin so that there is no build-up of lining to be shed as a 'period'.

Side effects are much lower than with other progestogens and the contraceptive effect can be an

Progestogen preparations

In place of a combined estrogen/progestogen preparation, the doctor may prescribe one of the estrogen-only preparations previously listed, together with any of the following progestogen preparations.

Tablets

Climanor (Resource Medical)
• Medroxyprogesterone acetate 5 mg

Provera (Pfizer)
• medroxyprogesterone acetate 2.5 mg, 5 mg or 10 mg

Caplets

Utrogestan (Marlborough Pharmaceuticals Ltd)
• progesterone 100 mg or 200 mg

Vaginal gel

Crinone (Serono)
• progesterone 8% (not licensed for HRT)

Intrauterine

Mirena (Bayer)
• Levonorgestrel 52 mg (20 micrograms per 24 hours)

advantage for women whose periods have not yet stopped. The main disadvantage is irregular bleeding but, for most women, periods stop completely.

Other prescription treatments
Tibolone

Tibolone (Livial) is a synthetic preparation of a type known as a selective tissue estrogenic activity regulator (STEAR). It is derived from plant sources and combines the properties of estrogen, progesterone and testosterone, in a single tablet.

It is taken continuously and is suitable for women whose periods have stopped. It is effective for treating vasomotor symptoms and reduces the risk of spine fractures. It may also improve sexual wellbeing. Tibolone is associated with a small increased risk of stroke in older, but not in younger, women. Most studies have shown a small increased risk of having endometrial cancer diagnosed with tibolone use. Limited data suggest that tibolone may be associated with a reduced risk of breast cancer.

However, in women who have had breast cancer in the past, tibolone appears to increase the risk of breast

Effectiveness of estrogen, estrogen/ progesterone and tibolone

Target symptom	Estrogen	Estrogen/ progestogen	Tibolone
Bone density	Improves symptoms	Improves symptoms	Improves symptoms
Flushes and sweats	Improves symptoms	Improves symptoms	Improves symptoms
Vaginal symptoms	Improves symptoms	Improves symptoms	Improves symptoms

The levonorgestrel intrauterine system (IUS)

The levonorgestrel intrauterine system (IUS) or Mirena is an effective contraceptive. It has a reservoir of progestogen that is slowly released directly into the uterus.

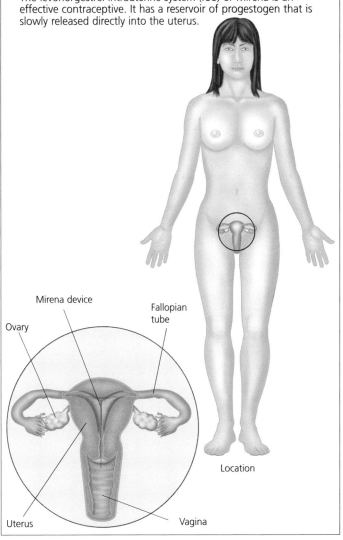

Mirena device

Fallopian tube

Ovary

Location

Uterus

Vagina

Advantages and disadvantages of different types of HRT

Advantages	Disadvantages
Tablets	
• Easy to take	• Unnatural delivery of hormone via the liver
• Easily reversible	• Must be taken every day
• Cheap	
• Can combine with progestogen	
Skin patches	
• Convenient	• Can become detached
• Easy to use	• Can irritate the skin
• More natural delivery of hormone into the bloodstream	• More expensive than tabl
• Easily reversible	• Must be changed once or twice a week
• Can combine with progestogen	
Gel	
• Easily reversible	• Must cover correct amou of skin
• Easy to use	• More expensive than tabl
• More natural delivery of hormone into the bloodstream	• Must use every day
	• If necessary, progestogen must be taken in a differe formulation

cancer recurrence. In younger women, the risk profile
of tibolone is broadly similar to that for conventional
combined HRT. For women aged more than about 60

Advantages and disadvantages of different types of HRT (contd)

dvantages	Disadvantages
nplants	
No missed doses	• Needs a small surgical procedure
More natural delivery of hormones into the bloodstream	• Can cause unnaturally high levels of hormones
Prolonged effect: 4–12 months	• Not rapidly reversible
Cheap	• Progestogen must be continued for some time after the final implant
aginal	
Useful if vaginal symptoms are the only problems	• Some types of estrogen are absorbed into the bloodstream
Easily reversible	• Progestogen may be necessary if used for longer than three months
	• Creams and pessaries can be messy

years, the risks associated with tibolone start to outweigh the benefits because of the increased risk of stroke.

Estrogen/progestogen combinations

These sex hormone therapies combine estrogen and progestogen

Brand	Estrogen	Dose
Climagest	Estradiol	1 or 2 mg
Clinorette	Estradiol	2 mg
Cyclo-Progynova	Estradiol	2 mg
Elleste Duet	Estradiol	1 or 2 mg
Evorel Sequi	Estradiol	50 µg
Femoston 1/10	Estradiol	1 mg
Femoston 2/10	Estradiol	2 mg
FemSeven Sequi	Estradiol	50 µg
Novofem	Estradiol	1 mg
Prempak-C	Conjugated estrogens	0.625 or 1.25 mg
Tridestra	Estradiol	2 mg
Trisequens	Estradiol	2 or 1 mg

Continuous estrogen/progestogen

These preparations combine estrogen and progestogen taken daily

Brand	Estrogen	Dose
Angeliq	Estradiol	1 mg
Climesse	Estradiol	2 mg
Elleste Duet Conti	Estradiol	2 mg
Evorel Conti	Estradiol	50 µg
Femoston Conti	Estradiol	0.5 or 1 mg
FemSeven Conti	Estradiol	50 µg
Indivina	Estradiol	1 or 2 mg
Kliofem	Estradiol	2 mg
Kliovance	Estradiol	1 mg
Nuvelle Continuous	Estradiol	2 mg
Premique	Conjugated estrogens	0.625 mg
Premique Low Dose	Conjugated estrogens	0.3 mg

and produce a monthly or quarterly bleed

Progestogen	Dose	Formulation	'Period'
Norethisterone	1 mg	Tablets	Monthly
Norethisterone	1 mg	Tablets	Monthly
Norgestrel	500 µg	Tablets	Monthly
Norethisterone	1 mg	Tablets	Monthly
Norethisterone	170 µg	Patches	Monthly
Dydrogesterone	10 mg	Tablets	Monthly
Dydrogesterone	10 mg	Tablets	Monthly
Levonorgestrel	10 µg	Patches	Monthly
Norethisterone	1 mg	Tablets	Monthly
Norgestrel	150 µg	Tablets	Monthly
Medroxyprogesterone	20 mg	Tablets	Quarterly
Norethisterone	1 mg	Tablets	Monthly

to avoid the need for a regular 'period'

Progestogen	Dose	Formulation	'Period'
Drospirenone	2 mg	Tablets	None
Norethisterone	0.7 mg	Tablets	None
Norethisterone	1 mg	Tablets	None
Norethisterone	170 µg	Patches	None
Dydrogesterone	2.5 or 5 mg	Tablets	None
Levonorgestrel	7 µg	Patches	None
Medroxyprogesterone	2.5 or 5 mg	Tablets	None
Norethisterone	1 mg	Tablets	None
Norethisterone	0.5 mg	Tablets	None
Norethisterone	1 mg	Tablets	None
Medroxyprogesterone	5 mg	Tablets	None
Medroxyprogesterone	1.5 mg	Tablets	None

Unopposed estrogen

If you have had a hysterectomy only estrogen treatment is necessary.

Brand	Estrogen	Dose	Formulation
Bedol	Estradiol	2 mg	Tablets
Climaval	Estradiol	1 or 2 mg	Tablets
Elleste Solo	Estradiol	1 or 2 mg	Tablets
Elleste Solo MX	Estradiol	40 or 80 µg	Patches
Estraderm MX	Estradiol	25, 50, 75 or 100 µg	Patches
Estradot	Estradiol	25, 37.5, 50, 75 or 100 µg	Patches
Evorel	Estradiol	25, 50, 75 or 100 µg	Patches
FemSeven	Estradiol	50, 75 or 100 µg	Patches
Hormonin	Estriol, estrone and estradiol	1 strength	Tablets
Oestrogel	Estradiol	1.5 mg	Gel
Premarin	Conjugated estrogens	0.3, 0.625 or 1.25 mg	Tablets
Progynova	Estradiol	1 or 2 mg	Tablets
Progynova TS	Estradiol	50 or 100 µg	Patches
Sandrena	Estradiol	0.5 or 1 mg	Gel
Zumenon	Estradiol	1 or 2 mg	Tablets

Local estrogen

Estrogen can be applied directly (locally) to the area producing symptoms, for example, dry vagina. Use them strictly as prescribed because the estrogen, if overused, can be absorbed through the skin into the bloodstream and affect the whole body.

Brand	Estrogen	Dose	Formulation
Estring	Estradiol	7.5 µg	Vaginal ring
Gynest	Estriol	0.01%	Vaginal cream
Ortho-Gynest	Estriol	0.5 mg	Vaginal pessary
Ovestin	Estriol	0.1%	Vaginal cream
Vagifem	Estradiol	10 µg	Vaginal tablets

Selective tissue estrogenic activity regulator (STEAR)

This preparation combines the properties of estrogen, progestogen and testosterone.

Brand	Drug	Dose	Formulation
Livial	Tibolone	2.5 mg	Tablets

KEY POINTS

■ There are different types of estrogen and progestogen and some types may not suit you

■ The hormones (estrogen and progestogen) are taken cyclically during the menopause but may be taken continuously once periods have stopped

■ In addition to tablets, estrogen is available as a patch, gel, vaginal ring or implant

■ Each of these ways of taking hormones has different advantages and disadvantages

■ Other more specific preparations are available, for example local estrogen for vaginal dryness and testosterone for loss of interest in sex

How to take HRT

The importance of progestogen

There are many different types of HRT. For women who have had a hysterectomy, most need take only estrogen, otherwise they need to take progestogen as well to protect them from cancer of the lining of the uterus. Sometimes women who have had a hysterectomy as a result of endometriosis are advised to take additional progestogens. Endometriosis occurs when the endometrium, the lining of the uterus, is found outside the uterus in other parts of the body. It is stimulated by estrogen and suppressed by progestogen – hence the benefits of the latter hormone.

Women with a uterus

Sequential combined HRT (cyclical)

This is estrogen combined with cyclical progestogen and is the HRT that most women use. Estrogen is taken continuously, without a break. It can be taken daily as a tablet, once or twice a week as a patch, or as a gel, vaginal ring or implant. Progestogen is added

Is HRT right for you?
You may find this flowchart useful to help with your choices.

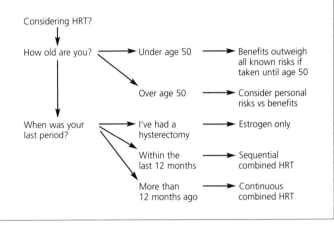

Considering HRT?

How old are you? → Under age 50 → Benefits outweigh all known risks if taken until age 50

Over age 50 → Consider personal risks vs benefits

When was your last period? → I've had a hysterectomy → Estrogen only

Within the last 12 months → Sequential combined HRT

More than 12 months ago → Continuous combined HRT

every month, either as a course of tablets lasting 10 to 14 days or as a combined patch with estrogen, replaced twice weekly.

Calendar packs are available to help remember when to take the progestogen. If estrogen and progestogen are prescribed separately, most doctors recommend that the progestogen course is started on the first day of every calendar month. All these forms of HRT should give a withdrawal bleed around or shortly after the end of the progestogen course. Any unexpected bleeding should be reported to the doctor.

More recently, long-cycle HRT has been introduced. This involves taking estrogen every day as usual, but taking the progestogen course only every three months. This means that there are only four withdrawal bleeds every year. A disadvantage of this regimen is that a relatively high dose of progestogen is needed, which

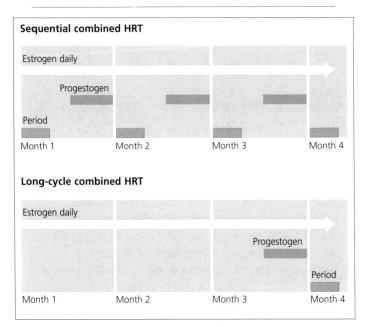

Sequential combined HRT

Estrogen daily

Progestogen

Period

Month 1   Month 2   Month 3   Month 4

Long-cycle combined HRT

Estrogen daily

Progestogen

Period

Month 1   Month 2   Month 3   Month 4

can give side effects such as bloating, headaches and irritability, as well as heavy and/or prolonged bleeding. Despite this, long-cycle HRT is useful for women whose natural periods are infrequent.

Continuous combined HRT

Most women who have gone through the menopause do not wish to return to monthly periods. To avoid this, a combination of estrogen and progestogen is taken daily (hence the term 'continuous combined HRT'). Taking both hormones together prevents any thickening of the uterine lining, making a withdrawal bleed unnecessary while providing protection against endometrial cancer. Although it can be taken by premenopausal women, irregular bleeding is a common problem.

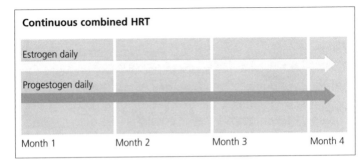

Even in postmenopausal women, unpredictable bleeding may occur during the first few months, sometimes heavy and prolonged. However, in most women who persevere, bleeding usually settles within 12 months. Bleeding is less likely the longer the woman has been postmenopausal before starting the treatment. So continuous combined HRT is generally recommended only if the woman has been postmenopausal for at least a year. In such cases, continuous combined HRT can be highly satisfactory, although missed pills can often lead to some spotting.

If you are postmenopausal and have been taking cyclical HRT but want to change to a period-free type, you should start your new tablets at the end of a withdrawal bleed, which is usually several days into a fresh pack of your old cyclical HRT. This reduces the likelihood of any unwanted bleeding, because your uterine lining is already thin when you start your new HRT.

A recent advance has been to give continuous estrogen to women who are using the progestogen-releasing intrauterine system, IUS (Mirena), used for contraception. This has a particular advantage for women who are at risk of pregnancy. It also keeps the uterine lining thin because the progestogen is released directly into the uterus and has few side effects. The IUS is also used to relieve painful or heavy periods. Although it is widely used together with estrogen for HRT, it is not currently licensed (see Glossary on page 148) for this indication in the UK. As with other period-free regimens, irregular bleeding can occur in the first few months but this usually settles quickly.

Cyclical estrogen

Estrogen treatment used to be given for three out of every four weeks, with no progestogen therapy to women with a uterus. But with this treatment, menopausal symptoms returned during the estrogen-free week and the risk of endometrial cancer is increased. It is no longer recommended in the UK, but is still prescribed in some other countries. Those women who take estrogen in this way should see a doctor and discuss other forms of HRT.

Women who have had a hysterectomy
Continuous estrogen

Women who have had a hysterectomy have the advantage of not needing to take progestogen. This reduces the likelihood of unwanted side effects. They can take daily estrogen tablets, once- or twice-weekly patches, daily gel, a three-monthly vaginal ring or six-monthly implants.

Women who have vaginal symptoms only
Local estrogen

Topical estrogen delivered directly into the vagina is very useful for local symptoms in the absence of other menopausal symptoms. They are available as creams, pessaries, tablets and a vaginal ring. Symptoms usually respond within three months of starting treatment but it can take up to a year of continuous use before a benefit is noticed. Most brands of vaginal estrogen result in very little absorption into the bloodstream so, if used short term (up to three months), no additional progestogen therapy is necessary. However, if conjugated equine estrogen cream is used, or if other local estrogen is used long term, additional progestogen may be necessary, unless the woman has had a hysterectomy. If she is using vaginal estrogen and experiences unexpected bleeding, she must see her doctor.

What is the right dose of HRT?
How much estrogen?
The dose of estrogen taken depends on the reason why it is being taken. Relief of severe symptoms requires a higher dose than relief of mild symptoms. Younger women also need higher doses to get the same benefit as older women. Many women wonder why their hormone levels are not tested – this is because normal estrogen levels vary so much that it is more appropriate to monitor symptom control. If symptoms are not adequately controlled, the dose of estrogen needs increasing; if side effects are a problem, the dose is too high. Research suggests that even low doses can protect against osteoporosis.

How much progestogen?
The dose of progestogen has to be high enough to eliminate the risk of cancer of the lining of the uterus (endometrial cancer) almost completely. However, unnecessarily high doses should be avoided because progestogen may increase the risk of breast cancer when taken with estrogen.

KEY POINTS

- Unless a woman has had a hysterectomy, she must use progestogen in addition to estrogen, in order to protect her uterine lining from cancer

- Women going through the menopause usually use sequential combined HRT, with a withdrawal bleed when they stop the progestogen each month

- Postmenopausal women can use continuous combined HRT and do not have to have periods

- The lowest dose of estrogen necessary to treat menopausal symptoms is recommended

HRT: when to start and when to stop

When should you start HRT?

The best time to start HRT depends on your personal circumstances, the likely balance of risks versus benefits and your personal preference. HRT is usually started around the menopause in order to control hot flushes and sweats. However, it can be started at any age, if there is good reason to do so.

How long should you take HRT for?

Most women take HRT for a couple of years, in order to treat menopausal symptoms. If taken for up to five years, there is no evidence that it increases the risk of breast cancer. Some women continue to have severe menopausal symptoms beyond five years. For these women HRT remains an effective option, particularly if non-hormonal treatments are not effective.

However, long-term use can be associated with increased risk of breast cancer and this is higher with combined HRT than with estrogen-only HRT. There is also an increased risk of venous thrombosis and stroke. Most of these risks increase with increasing age anyway, not just with HRT use. Only you can decide whether the benefits of HRT outweigh these potential risks. Your decision will depend on how troublesome your menopausal symptoms are to you.

Women in their 60s or older who need treatment to prevent osteoporosis are usually advised to consider non-hormonal treatments first. Some women prefer to choose HRT. However, in order to prevent osteoporosis, life-long treatment is necessary because bone loss begins as soon as HRT is stopped.

Some women wish to continue HRT lifelong, just because it makes them feel so well. There is no reason why they should not do this, provided that the benefit is carefully weighed against the risk.

Women who have had a premature menopause, either spontaneously or through surgical removal of the ovaries, are, we understand at present, at no additional risk from HRT use when taken until they are 50, no matter for how many years they take it. This is because HRT is replacing the hormones that would normally be produced until the natural menopause.

How do you stop HRT?

HRT maintains a hormonal balance, levelling out the hormonal fluctuations that are responsible for menopausal symptoms. Stopping HRT suddenly will provoke an abrupt drop in estrogen and symptoms return. When this happens, the symptoms result from the sudden change in HRT and do not necessarily reflect what is happening with your own hormones.

To avoid this, and to enable you to assess whether or not menopausal symptoms caused by your own hormones have abated, you should gradually reduce the estrogen dose over a period of two to six months, typically by cutting pills or matrix patches (patches will not leak if cut) into increasingly smaller doses or using increasingly smaller amounts of gel. This allows the level to decline gradually, minimising the likelihood of symptoms developing. You must continue to take the same progestogen dose, in the usual way, until you have completely stopped the estrogen.

Women using estrogen implants can also gradually reduce the dose of each implant when it is replaced every six months. However, the effects of an implant on the uterine lining can continue for up to two to three years. So, unless the woman has had a hysterectomy, she must continue taking progestogen until the implant has worn off. This can be assessed by whether or not a withdrawal bleed occurs following a course of progestogen. If it does, then estrogen is still present, causing the lining of the uterus to thicken. If there is no bleeding, it is usually safe to stop taking progestogen.

KEY POINTS

■ HRT can be started at any age but is most often started around the menopause to control flushes and sweats

■ If taken for up to five years beyond the menopause, there are no major risks

■ HRT can be taken lifelong but using it for more than five years carries increased risks

■ Women who have a premature menopause should take HRT until they are 50; this is not associated with any increased risks because it is replacing hormones that would have normally been present

■ Suddenly stopping HRT can result in the return of flushes and sweats resulting from a sudden drop in estrogen – this can be minimised by reducing the estrogen dose over several months

Side effects of HRT

Resolving side effects

Around 35 per cent of women stop taking HRT because of unwanted side effects. Often, these side effects could be resolved by a change in the dose or type of HRT. So it is very important to discuss feelings and experiences with the doctor before just stopping HRT. If a woman decides to stop, she should talk to her doctor about how best to do this (see previous chapter).

Side effects of estrogen

Fluid retention, bloating, breast tenderness, nausea, leg cramps and gastric upset are symptoms associated with high levels of estrogen, and are not uncommon when starting HRT. If they have not settled by the end of the third month from starting HRT, it is worth considering lowering your estrogen dose or changing to a different form of HRT.

Leg cramps can improve with exercise and regular stretching of the calf muscles. Gastric upsets usually improve if oral HRT is taken with food. Breast tenderness is sometimes alleviated by a low-fat, low-carbohydrate diet. Evening primrose oil can also help.

Side effects of progestogen

Side effects are much more common with cyclical courses than with continuous progestogen. The most common problem is 'premenstrual' symptoms, which affect up to 20 per cent of women taking cyclical progestogen. These symptoms include fluid retention, breast tenderness, mood swings, depression, acne, lower abdominal pains and backache. They are most apparent when starting HRT and often resolve with continued use.

If they persist, altering the dose or type of progestogen can help. Changing the route of delivery can also help – for example, from tablets to patches.

If symptoms are particularly severe, the progestogen course could be taken every three months rather than

Side effects of estrogen and progestogen

Estrogen and progestogen are associated with a number of side effects. Some of the most frequently occurring side effects that women may experience when they start HRT are listed below. Many resolve within the first two to three months.

Estrogen

- Fluid retention
- Feeling of bloatedness
- Breast tenderness
- Nausea
- Stomach upset
- Leg cramps

Progestogen

- Fluid retention
- Breast tenderness
- Depression
- Nausea
- Irritability
- Headaches
- Mood swings
- Abdominal pain
- Backache
- Acne

monthly. Alternatively, the duration of the progestogen could be shortened, but reducing the course to less than ten days reduces the protective effect against cancer of the lining of the uterus and can provoke irregular bleeding.

Postmenopausal women can change to continuous combined HRT, which requires a lower dose of progestogen than cyclical regimens and has the advantage of being period free.

Other side effects of HRT
Bleeding
Unless you have had a hysterectomy, you will probably need cyclical progestogen, taken as a course, usually as tablets or patches, every month. If you are taking cyclical progestogen, a withdrawal bleed or 'period' usually starts around the end of the progestogen course.

It is useful to keep a record of when you use the progestogen and when your period starts. If your bleeding starts early in the progestogen course or if you get bleeding unexpectedly at other times of the month, you should report this to your doctor. It is quite common in the first few months of taking HRT, but if unusual bleeding starts after taking HRT for six months or longer, the cause needs to be assessed.

Investigating suspicious bleeding
You may only need to change the dose, timing, duration or type of progestogen but your doctor may want to check that the progestogen is providing adequate protection against cancerous changes developing in the uterus.

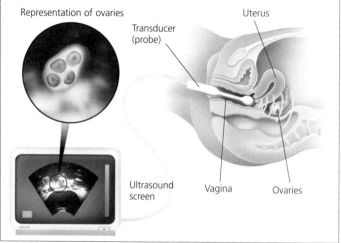

Transvaginal ultrasound scan
During a transvaginal ultrasound scan (TVS) a small probe is inserted into the vagina and the ultrasound waves create a picture of the uterus and ovaries.

Representation of ovaries

Uterus

Transducer (probe)

Ultrasound screen

Vagina

Ovaries

Transvaginal ultrasound scan
In many gynaecology departments, one of the first steps after a manual internal examination has been done is to arrange for you to have a transvaginal ultrasound scan (TVS). A small probe (transducer) is inserted into the vagina and the ultrasound waves create a picture of the uterus and ovaries. A TVS can also be used to measure the thickness of the endometrium and identify common benign causes of bleeding such as fibroids or polyps. Rarely cancer of the lining of the uterus may be a cause.

Endometrial biopsy
Some doctors perform an endometrial biopsy. This involves taking a small sample of the lining of the uterus. It can be done in the outpatient department,

Endometrial biopsy

During an endometrial biopsy a small sample is taken from the lining of the uterus.

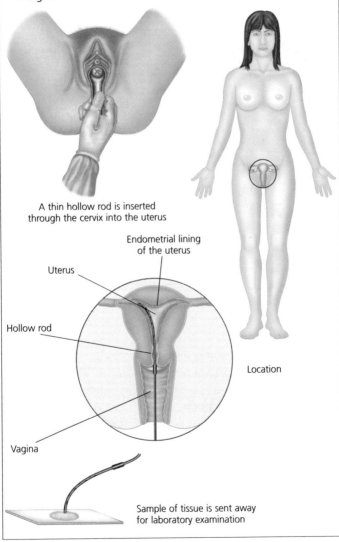

A thin hollow rod is inserted through the cervix into the uterus

Endometrial lining of the uterus

Uterus

Hollow rod

Vagina

Location

Sample of tissue is sent away for laboratory examination

without the need for an anaesthetic, and you can go home immediately after. A thin hollow rod is inserted through your cervix, into the uterus. A small sample of tissue is then scraped from the endometrial lining of the uterus. You may feel some cramping pains but these usually pass very quickly. It is usual for some spotting to occur for a few hours after.

Hysteroscopy
Most hospitals can now perform a hysteroscopy in the outpatient department. Although this investigation has the advantage of enabling the doctor to look directly

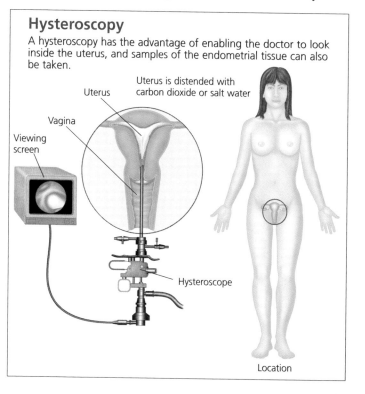

Hysteroscopy

A hysteroscopy has the advantage of enabling the doctor to look inside the uterus, and samples of the endometrial tissue can also be taken.

Uterus is distended with carbon dioxide or salt water

Uterus

Vagina

Viewing screen

Hysteroscope

Location

Investigating suspicious bleeding

Unexpected bleeding may be an indication of an underlying problem needing specific treatment and is usually investigated by one of the following techniques.

Technique	Anaesthetic required?
• *Endometrial biopsy:* taking a sample of the lining of the uterus using a narrow hollow rod	No
• *Transvaginal ultrasound scan (TVS):* a small probe is inserted into the vagina to view the uterus and ovaries	No
• *Hysteroscopy:* a camera is inserted into the uterus to look at the endometrium and enable direct samples of the tissue to be taken	Sometimes

at the endometrium, it is a longer procedure than a TVS or endometrial biopsy. A long thin rod with a video camera and a light attached to it is inserted into the uterus. The uterus is distended slightly by pumping in carbon dioxide gas or saline (salt water), allowing the doctor to look at the endometrium. Small scissors can be inserted through the rod to take samples. By using local anaesthesia, there is usually minimal discomfort during hysteroscopy. Most women are able to get up and return to their normal activities immediately, although mild cramps and some bloody discharge may occur for a day or two.

Weight gain

Although many women are concerned that HRT will make them put on weight, studies show that HRT users often gain less weight than non-users after the menopause. A few women are sensitive to oral estrogen, particularly if the dose is too high, causing them to retain fluid and gain weight. Simply reducing the dose or changing to a non-oral form can resolve this.

Headaches

Fluctuating hormone levels can trigger migraine and headaches. These fluctuations are common with oral forms of HRT (taken by mouth). Switching to a non-oral form (for example, patches) may solve the problem.

KEY POINTS

■ Side effects are common when starting HRT but most resolve in the first two to three months

■ If side effects persist, they must be discussed with a doctor because there are various ways to minimise them

■ Often side effects can be resolved by a change in dose or type of HRT

■ One way is to try a lower dose of progestogen but it must be enough to protect from endometrial cancer

■ A different route of delivery may relieve side effects – for example, change from tablets to patches

■ Seek medical advice if you have any abnormal bleeding

HRT: who can and who can't take it

Who can take HRT?

There are very few conditions that prevent women from using HRT. However, there is often some misinformation about who can and who can't take it.

Women with any of the following conditions can use HRT, although some may need specialist supervision:

- Cervical cancer
- Coeliac disease (non-oral route preferred)
- Crohn's disease (non-oral route preferred)
- Diabetes
- Epilepsy
- High blood pressure (non-oral route preferred)
- High cholesterol (route depends on lipid profile)
- Kidney failure
- Mild liver disease (non-oral route preferred)
- Malignant melanoma

- Migraine (non-oral route preferred)
- Ovarian cancer
- Parkinson's disease
- Rheumatoid arthritis
- Thyroid disease
- Heart valve disease.

Who should be cautious about HRT?
Benign breast lumps
There is no convincing evidence that this condition is associated with a greater than expected risk of breast cancer in women using HRT. If a woman has breast lumps, she should be checked before starting HRT to make sure that they are not cancerous. Regular checks should be continued once treatment has begun.

Endometriosis
Sometimes the tissue that lines the uterus is found in abnormal sites such as the rectum or navel. In the same way that the lining of the uterus is shed each month during menstruation, these other sites also bleed, causing severe pain and heavy periods. This condition, known as endometriosis, is stimulated by estrogen and improves with the menopause.

HRT can occasionally reactivate the condition so if you have had endometriosis you should be cautious when taking HRT, monitoring any symptoms, particularly of pain on intercourse and heavy or irregular bleeding. Even if you have had a hysterectomy, some doctors will recommend that you take continuous progestogen to prevent the endometriosis recurring. This is because the lining of the uterus cannot grow in the presence of progestogen.

Fibroids

Fibroids (non-cancerous growths in the muscle of the uterus) are very common. They are sensitive to estrogen so they often grow during pregnancy as the level of estrogen in the body rises, and shrink after the menopause. As a result of this, fibroids can enlarge with HRT, causing heavy withdrawal bleeding. Continuous progestogen can reduce the likelihood of fibroids increasing in size. The levonorgestrel intrauterine system (see page 86) is sometimes used to help treat fibroids.

Gallstones

If you have gallstones you should discuss HRT use with your doctor because the gallstones may enlarge, particularly with oral therapy. If you have had problems with gallstones in the past, some doctors suggest that you should use patches or implants rather than tablets to reduce the amount of estrogen passing through the liver. It is safe to use HRT if you have had an operation to remove gallstones.

Otosclerosis

Otosclerosis is an inherited cause of hearing loss resulting from the growth of extra bone which prevents the small bones in the ear from working properly. This condition can deteriorate rapidly during pregnancy, suggesting a link with estrogen. HRT may have the same effect, so specialist advice should be sought before starting treatment.

Who should not take HRT?
Breast cancer

There are two main types of breast cancers – those that

are sensitive to estrogen and those that are not. If you have been successfully treated for non-estrogen-dependent breast cancer you may still be able to take HRT, particularly if you have a specific reason to do so – such as relieving severe hot flushes. However, you need to be carefully supervised by a specialist. Even women with estrogen-dependent cancers can usually take vaginal estrogen to treat local symptoms.

Endometrial cancer

The majority of women found to have endometrial cancer are likely to be cured by hysterectomy. Following successful surgery, many women subsequently develop debilitating menopausal symptoms, which may not always respond to non-hormonal treatment. If a woman with a history of endometrial cancer develops symptoms that warrant HRT, it can usually be prescribed. However, because endometrial cancer is estrogen dependent, most doctors prescribe progestogen as well as estrogen in order to minimise the likelihood of recurrence.

Severe liver disease

You should not take HRT if you have jaundice as a result of severe liver disease. This is because most of the estrogen, particularly if taken by mouth, is broken down by your liver, increasing its metabolic load. This is not a problem for a healthy liver but a diseased liver may not be able to cope with this extra workload. If your jaundice improves and your liver works normally again, then there is no reason why HRT should not be taken. Non-oral forms – patches or implants – are recommended because lower hormone levels pass through the liver.

Blood clots (venous thrombosis)

Venous thrombosis can result from an underlying genetic condition or a blood clotting disorder (thrombophilia). If you have a close family member who had an unexplained blood clot under the age of 45, investigations to screen for thrombophilia or underlying disease may be necessary before HRT can be considered.

Heart attacks and strokes

It is not recommended that you should start HRT in order to try to prevent heart attacks or strokes if you have already experienced one. However, if you have a history of either of these, you may be given HRT if you have severe menopausal symptoms or are at risk of osteoporosis. If you have had a heart attack or stroke and are already taking HRT, this may not be a reason to stop it.

Pregnancy

Despite fertility being low as women approach the menopause, it is still possible to become pregnant. Most HRTs are not contraceptive. Women who have taken HRT and then found that they are pregnant can be reassured that it is unlikely that HRT will adversely affect outcome of pregnancy. However, miscarriage rates are high in older women for other reasons.

Undiagnosed vaginal bleeding

HRT should not be used to control unusual bleeding until the cause of the bleeding has been assessed. This is because HRT itself can cause unexpected bleeding and mask an underlying problem that may need treatment.

KEY POINTS

■ Few women are unable to take HRT on medical grounds

■ HRT is not recommended if you have estrogen-dependent cancers such as cancer of the endometrium or estrogen-dependent breast cancer

■ You should not start HRT while you have venous thrombosis or active liver disease

■ If you experience unexplained vaginal bleeding, seek medical advice

Controlling symptoms without HRT

Although HRT is the 'gold standard' for controlling menopausal symptoms, relieving up to 80 per cent of hot flushes, not every woman can, needs to or wants to take it. For many women, particularly those with mild symptoms, one or other of the following options can be effective.

Controlling hot flushes using non-prescription remedies

Many women use non-prescription remedies to treat hot flushes, such as isoflavones. Also popular are dong quai, evening primrose oil, vitamin E, ginseng, liquorice and natural progesterone creams. Most of these are classed as dietary supplements and so are not regulated in the same way as drugs. Hence these treatments can be sold in health shops, supermarkets and pharmacies without evidence that they are either effective or safe.

Also, information about how they interact with other therapies and prescription drugs is often limited and they may have serious side effects.

Isoflavones

These plant estrogens are often called phytoestrogens. Two common sources of isoflavones are soy and red clover. The potential for toxic or adverse side effects with these doses is minimal but, because of their potential hormonal effects, they should not be used by women with a history of breast cancer. Although clinical trials have suggested that isoflavones can alleviate hot flushes, placebo tablets were just as effective.

Black cohosh

Preparations made from the thick underground stems (rhizomes) of the herb black cohosh have been studied, with varying reports of efficacy. Almost all the studies have used different formulations and doses, so the results are difficult to compare. Although a popular remedy, black cohosh is not recommended because there have been reports of toxic effects on the liver.

Dong quai

This herb is commonly used in traditional Chinese medicine to treat gynaecological problems. Studies using the herb to control hot flushes have shown little benefit. Women using warfarin should not take dong quai.

Evening primrose oil

Although very effective for treating breast tenderness premenstrually, even high doses of evening primrose oil (two grams daily) have shown little benefit for hot flushes. Side effects include nausea and diarrhoea.

Vitamin E
Studies using vitamin E in doses up to 400 IU twice daily have not shown much effect on hot flushes. Side effects are few and not serious.

Ginseng
Studies with ginseng have not shown benefit on hot flushes. Ginseng can adversely interact with monoamine oxidase inhibitors (MAOIs), which may be prescribed for treatment of depression, and with anticoagulants such as aspirin and warfarin.

Liquorice
The root of the liquorice plant is used in many Chinese preparations for menopausal symptoms. However, there are no studies to show either safety or efficacy. Women taking diuretics should not use liquorice. High doses of liquorice can cause fluid retention and high blood pressure.

Natural progesterone cream
Progesterone is synthesised by a chemical process from plants such as soy beans or wild yam. Some of the products contain progesterone indistinguishable from a woman's own natural progesterone. Others contain only chemical precursors of progesterone found in plants, which are inactive in humans because they cannot be converted to progesterone. As these creams are regulated as dietary supplements, it is not possible to know which products are which.

Although creams containing progesterone, often combined with vitamin E and aloe vera, have shown a positive effect on flushes there are safety concerns about unregulated hormonal treatments. Women using estrogen replacement therapy should not use progesterone creams in place of prescribed progestogens (synthetic progesterones), because they may not protect the endometrium.

Reducing hot flushes using prescription drugs but without hormonal treatment

Some women prefer first to try non-prescription and non-hormonal remedies to control hot flushes. These include herbal and homoeopathic options. If these do not work, women should ask their GPs to consider which of the non-hormonal prescriptions (in other words not HRT) are suitable for them.

Serotonin inhibitors

Serotonin is a neurotransmitter in the brain and is important in the control of mood and behaviour, feeding and hunger, temperature regulation and sleep. Selective serotonin reuptake inhibitors (SSRIs) are licensed for the treatment of depression. Depression is caused by low serotonin levels and SSRIs increase the serotonin levels. However, research has also shown that lower doses of SSRIs are effective for a wide variety of other conditions, including control of chronic pain conditions, migraine and hot flushes. The three most commonly used for hot flushes are venlafaxine (Efexor), paroxetine (Seroxat) and fluoxetine (Prozac). Trials suggest that there can be up to a 60 per cent reduction in flushes. Although symptoms can improve immediately, it may take up to eight weeks before any benefit is seen. The most common side effects are nausea, weight loss and reduced sex drive.

Gabapentin

This drug is licensed for the control of epilepsy but is also used for chronic pain conditions. and can halve the rate of hot flushes. Side effects include dizziness and feeling light-headed as well as some fluid retention and tiredness. As antacids (indigestion remedies) can reduce the amount of gabapentin that gets into the body, gabapentin should be taken at least two hours after an antacid is used.

Clonidine

This drug, originally developed for the treatment of high blood pressure, can alleviate mild hot flushes but is less effective than SSRIs or gabapentin. Side effects of drowsiness, dizziness, constipation and depression are common.

Reducing hot flushes using prescription hormone treatment that is not HRT
Combined oral contraceptives (see page 130)

Combined oral contraceptives (COCs), containing synthetic estrogen (ethinylestradiol) and synthetic progesterone (progestogen), inhibit ovulation. Healthy, non-smoking women can take low-dose COCs right up to the menopause. They provide contraception and prevent hot flushes but the doses of hormones are much higher than HRT. This means that the risk of blood clots is greater than for HRT but benefits, particularly of lighter menstrual periods, can make COCs a good option for some women.

Progestogen (see pages 130–2)

Although progestogen is usually taken together with estrogen for HRT, high-dose progestogen can be effective on its own. Depot medroxyprogesterone acetate or DMPA (Depo-Provera) can be given by injection every three months and also provides contraception.

The side effects can include weight gain and irregular bleeding. There is also some controversy about the effect of injectable DMPA on bone density. Medroxyprogesterone tablets, 20 mg a day, are also effective and result in less irregular bleeding. It can take up to six weeks to reach its maximum effect. Another progestogen tablet, megestrol acetate, 20 mg twice a day, is also effective.

KEY POINTS

- HRT is the most effective treatment for menopausal symptoms

- There is little evidence to show that non-prescription dietary supplements and herbal remedies are any more effective than placebo treatments

- For women who cannot or do not wish to take HRT, venlafaxine, paroxetine, fluoxetine or gabapentin is a non-hormonal option available on prescription

Contraception around the menopause

Do I need contraception?

Women approaching the menopause often wrongly assume that they no longer need to use contraception. It is certainly true that a woman in her 40s is about half as fertile as a woman in her 20s. Also, her eggs are of a poorer quality and ovulation is less regular, until she finally stops ovulating and experiences the menopause. Despite this, pregnancy can occur. If you are not protected and your periods suddenly stop, you might assume it is the menopause, but it could be that you are pregnant.

Although many babies born to older mothers are very healthy, genetic abnormalities such as Down's syndrome become more common. The risk of miscarriage and risks to mother and baby are also increased in older women. Therefore effective contraception can be as important for a woman in her late 40s as it is for a woman in her teens or 20s.

Contraception should be continued for at least 12 months after the last period in women over the age of 50. Women who have an earlier menopause are advised to continue contraception for at least two years after the last period.

Hormonal contraception
Combined hormonal contraceptives

Combined oral contraceptives (COCs; commonly known as the pill), the contraceptive patch and the contraceptive vaginal ring contain both synthetic estrogen and progestogen. They work by inhibiting ovulation. In addition to their contraceptive effects, they will also provide relief from menopausal symptoms. Healthy, non-smoking women can use modern, low-dose, combined hormonal contraceptives until one or two years after the menopause. Although synthetic estrogens increase the risk of blood clots, this has to be balanced against potential health benefits for perimenopausal women including relief of premenstrual symptoms and regular periods that are less painful and heavy than natural periods. There is also some evidence that combined oral contraceptives have a positive effect on bone density.

Progestogen-only methods

Although postmenopausal use of progestogen is associated with increased risk of breast cancer, there is no evidence of this effect when progestogens are taken before the menopause. The advantage of progestogen-only methods over combined hormonal contraception is that there is no associated increased risk of blood clots with the former. There are several types of contraception that contain just progestogen.

Each of them works in a slightly different way. Progestogen-only methods can be prescribed to many women at risk of blood clots who cannot use combined hormonal contraceptives, including smokers.

Progestogen-only pill

The progestogen-only pill (POP), also known as the mini-pill, is taken every day and contains a very low dose of progestogen. Unlike COCs, which inhibit ovulation, standard POPs have minimal effect on ovulation but act by thickening cervical mucus and preventing sperm getting into the uterus. For women over 35, standard POPs are as effective as combined oral contraceptives. A newer POP, called Cerazette, does inhibit ovulation. The main potential problem with POPs is irregular bleeding. This may be resolved by changing to a different type of POP. In contrast, some women find that their periods stop.

Injectables

There are two types of progestogen that can be injected: depot medroxyprogesterone acetate (DMPA; Depo-Provera) and norethisterone acetate (NETA; Noristerat). As with the combined pill, they work by inhibiting the monthly release of the egg from the ovaries. Both types are administered by health-care professionals by deep intramuscular injection into the buttock or upper arm: DMPA every twelve weeks and NETA every eight weeks. Injectables can relieve premenstrual symptoms and heavy, painful periods. They can be associated with weight gain and irregular bleeding, although this usually resolves with continued use.

Implants

Implanon is a single rod, about the size of a hairgrip, which contains progestogen. It works by switching off the normal menstrual cycle, similar to the combined pill and injectables. A trained health-care professional injects the rod just under the skin on the inner side of the upper arm. It is both palpable and visible after insertion but is a highly effective contraceptive, lasting for up to three years.

It is not licensed (see Glossary, page 148) for use in women aged over 40, although you can use it if you and your doctor think that it is a suitable method for you. Implants can relieve many period-related problems, particularly heavy, painful periods. The main drawbacks can be weight gain and irregular bleeding, which can be frequent or prolonged in up to 20 per cent of users.

Levonorgestrel intrauterine system

The levonorgestrel intrauterine system (Mirena) is a small T-shaped device containing progestogen inserted into the uterus by trained health-care professionals. Progestogen is released directly into the uterus, keeping the uterine lining or endometrium thin (important for lower risk of endometrial cancer). Side effects are few as the hormonal effect is essentially within the uterus, and only small amounts of hormone reach the bloodstream. The IUS is as effective as sterilisation but is easily reversed by removal of the device. It is also an effective treatment for heavy, painful periods. In addition to its use as a contraceptive, the IUS can also be used together with natural estrogen supplements as HRT. Occasionally, irregular, frequent or prolonged bleeding can necessitate removal of the device.

Non-hormonal contraception
Sterilisation
Both vasectomy and female sterilisation are popular in older couples. However, sterilisation needs to be considered very carefully because this method is essentially irreversible. Many reversible methods such as the IUS and implants are as effective as sterilisation, often with added benefits for period-related problems.

Copper intrauterine device
Modern intrauterine devices (IUDs), often called coils, offer highly effective reversible contraception. They contain copper, which kills sperm before they can reach the uterus. If inserted after your fortieth birthday, an IUD can remain in place until after your menopause. The main disadvantage of this method is increased menstrual blood loss and period pains, so it is not recommended if you already have heavy or painful periods.

Barrier methods
Barrier methods can be sufficiently effective in older women because their fertility is lower. Condoms (including the female condom Femidom) are the most popular barrier method and are widely available without prescription. Polyurethane condoms are available for those with latex allergy. Diaphragms are popular with many couples and new female barrier methods are now available over the counter.

Vaginal sponge
A small, one-size, single-use, disposable vaginal sponge is available over the counter. It is impregnated with three different spermicides. In addition to the effects of

the spermicides, the sponge forms a physical barrier over the cervix and absorbs sperm.

Spermicides
In women over age 50, a spermicide can be sufficient on its own because fertility is so low. It can also help vaginal lubrication.

Coitus interruptus
Coitus interruptus or the withdrawal method is not a reliable contraceptive at any age and you should consider other more effective methods.

Fertility awareness
Methods such as measuring changes in temperature, checking cervical secretions and calculating the 'safe period' can be very effective for motivated women with regular menstrual periods. These methods become less reliable during the menopause as periods become erratic.

When can you stop using contraception?
If you are over 50, contraception can be stopped one year after your periods end. If you are under 50 and your periods stop, you should continue using contraception for another two years after what you believe to be the last period, provided that your periods do not return in that time. Barrier methods, spermicides alone or the contraceptive sponge should be sufficient at these times because your fertility is low.

As most women's natural periods stop around the age of 50, it is generally advisable to stop hormonal contraception when you are about that age and change to alternative contraception until you know that you are past the menopause.

HRT and contraception

HRT does not restore fertility, nor is it always an effective contraceptive. Therefore, if you start HRT before your periods have stopped naturally, there is a risk of pregnancy.

Most standard HRT methods are not contraceptive so additional non-hormonal contraception is usually recommended. One HRT regimen increasingly recommended is to use the progestogen-containing contraceptive IUS (Mirena) in conjunction with estrogen.

Withdrawal bleeds associated with some types of HRT can make it difficult to assess the timing of your natural menopause. Blood tests (see pages 10–11) can be taken in the estrogen-only phase of the sequential combined HRT and may sometimes indicate the menopause, but it is usually necessary to stop HRT to achieve a valid result. Otherwise contraception should be continued until you are 55 when it is safe to assume that you are no longer fertile.

KEY POINTS

■ Contraception is important if you are at risk of becoming pregnant

■ Most standard methods of HRT are not contraceptive so additional non-hormonal contraception may be necessary

■ Some hormonal methods of contraception also provide HRT

■ Contraception can be stopped two years after your last natural period if you are under 50, and one year after your last natural period if you are over 50

■ If you don't want to stop HRT to find out if you have gone through the menopause you should continue contraception until you are 55

HRT: conclusions

HRT has been available to women for over 60 years but for much of that time guidance for prescription has been based on biased observational studies. This has led to the false belief that HRT is a panacea for all age-related ailments in women.

Now we are fortunate to have the results from well-designed studies comparing HRT with inactive treatment, enabling us to assess more accurately the true benefits and risks of HRT. From these studies we see that certain types of HRT, notably standard dose conjugated oral estrogens, taken together with the progestogen medroxyprogesterone acetate, when given to postmenopausal women, can increase the risk of stroke, heart disease, venous thrombosis and breast cancer. Standard dose oral estrogen-only HRT can increase the risk of venous thrombosis and stroke but does not appear to increase the risk of breast cancer. All studies confirm the benefits of HRT on treating menopause symptoms, reducing the risk of fractures of the hip and spine, and of colorectal cancer.

On the basis of these results, recent recommendations for HRT have been amended to ensure that women are most likely to benefit from the prescription with minimal risks. Hence HRT remains an effective treatment for menopause symptoms.

Current recommendations correctly endorse that HRT should be prescribed on an individual basis and for the shortest time necessary. This is not defined by an arbitrary time limit but depends on the individual needs of the woman, who is fully informed about the pros and cons of HRT.

Although guidelines based on accurate evidence are laudable, it is important to recognise that much still remains unknown about HRT given to populations different from those included in published studies. Trials produce generalised statistics of the risks and benefits of a particular treatment given to a particular population, whereas a woman seeking help for severe menopausal symptoms wants to know how HRT is going to affect her. We still need information from well-designed studies assessing younger perimenopausal women taking HRT, particularly those with symptoms or those who are at high risk of osteoporosis. Furthermore, we need information about the risks and benefits of different types and doses of HRT: natural human estrogens are not the same as conjugated equine estrogens; non-oral routes may have different effects from tablets; and lower doses of estrogen may have the same benefits as higher doses but with less risk.

Future research will help further to define the role of HRT and will also herald safe and effective alternatives to HRT. In the meantime, if you are taking or considering taking HRT, it is sensible to take the lowest effective dose of hormones and reassess your continuing need at least annually.

Questions and answers

My breasts feel lumpy all over. How can I tell if a lump is cancer?

Breast tissue is affected by the different hormones produced during the menstrual cycle and also by HRT hormones. Many women notice that their breasts feel generally lumpy, particularly just before a period, without there being anything wrong. Getting to know what is normal for you and being aware of changes in your breasts is very important. You should look for changes in the outline or shape of the breast as you move your arms or lift the breast. Other changes to note are puckering or dimpling of the skin, changes in the nipple, or any lumps that you can see or feel.

If you find anything that worries you, check with your doctor without delay. In most cases, breast lumps are simple fluid-filled cysts and are not the result of cancer. However, if cancer is present, provided that it is treated early, it can often be cured.

Since the menopause, I feel tired most of the time, have lost interest in sex and feel generally low. Can HRT help?

Symptoms of depression are common in the years around the menopause, so it is not surprising that hormones are blamed. Hot flushes and night sweats can disrupt your sleep leading to loss of energy and low mood. By treating the flushes and sweats, HRT can certainly help you to get the best out of life again.

However, depressive symptoms can result from many other significant events that occur at much the same time as the menopause – children leaving home, separation or divorce, and illness or death of parents. Depression resulting from events such as these will not respond to HRT.

If you have menopausal symptoms that are a problem, it is certainly worth trying HRT. If your flushes and sweats improve but you are still feeling low, it is unlikely that hormones are the cause and you need to look for other reasons. Some women may need both HRT and antidepressants at this time.

My doctor has just started me on HRT. I was expecting to have blood tests or something to check my hormone levels but I was just asked lots of questions, given a prescription and told to make an appointment for three months' time. Don't I need any tests?

Hormone levels vary considerably and do not provide as much information as the symptoms you are experiencing. So your doctor is far more likely to ask questions than do tests! You will also be asked about your own and your family's medical history to ensure that it is safe for you to take HRT. If you are up to date with smear tests and mammograms, your doctor will not need to examine your breasts or do an internal examination, unless you have certain symptoms.

Once you have started HRT, you will usually be seen three months later to make sure that the type of HRT is right for you and to sort out any problem or concerns that you may have. When you are settled on HRT, you need only annual check-ups. However, if you have any concerns you should make an early appointment for review.

Most of the studies recently reported have been about one particular type of HRT. Do the results apply to all types of HRT or just this one?

Many of the recent studies about the long-term risk of HRT relate to one type of estrogen (conjugated equine estrogen) and one type of progestogen (medroxyprogesterone acetate or MPA). In the UK, products containing these hormones are tablets called Premarin, Premique and Premique Cycle.

It is impossible to know if the long-term risks shown in these studies also apply to HRT using estradiol and different progestogens. Clinical trials using different hormones and different routes of delivery are under way.

My mother shrank as she got older and was told that her spine was collapsing because her bones had got thin. What can I do to prevent the same happening to me?

Your natural build, how much exercise you take and your diet will provide some indication of how likely you are to be affected. Thin women, who take little exercise and avoid dairy products, are particularly at risk, especially if they smoke. As estrogen protects bone, the menopause, with decreasing levels of estrogen, represents an additional risk factor.

Your doctor may send you for a bone density scan to assess your baseline bone density before considering treatment. If you are experiencing menopausal symptoms and are at risk of osteoporosis, you may be offered HRT. Otherwise, non-hormonal treatments available on prescription such as the bisphosphonates are the first choice to prevent osteoporosis in older women.

I am 46 and my periods are very erratic but I'm not getting any other symptoms. Could this be the start of the menopause?

The first symptom of the 'change' or menopause is often a change in the pattern of periods, as you describe. Typically, periods will become more frequent and then they come further apart. You may skip one or two periods between otherwise regular cycles.

For some women, their periods cease with very few other symptoms. For others, flushes and sweats at first happen just in the week before a period and gradually become more frequent. Most women have had their last menstrual period by the time they are 54.

I've heard all about a type of HRT called Evista (raloxifene). What is it?

Raloxifene is not a natural hormone but is the first of a new class of synthetic compounds known as selective estrogen receptor modulators (SERMs). These mimic the protective actions of estrogen on bone without the unwanted effects on the lining of the uterus and breast tissue.

Clinical trials have shown that raloxifene can increase bone density, although not as well as conventional HRT. Raloxifene also seems to reduce the levels of cholesterol in the blood but there is no proof that this means that the risk of heart disease is reduced. Raloxifene also appears to protect against breast cancer. However, much larger clinical trials are necessary to confirm this early finding.

On the negative side, raloxifene carries a similar risk of venous thrombosis (blood clots in the legs and lungs) as HRT. It does not affect menopausal symptoms and may even cause hot flushes. Overall, it has limited use in management of the menopause but may be useful for postmenopausal women at risk of osteoporosis who cannot take bisphosphonates or HRT.

At 54 my periods stopped and I was lucky to have very few menopausal symptoms. But I'm now 57 and still experiencing severe hot flushes. I would like to try HRT but I have read that I would have to have periods again. Is this true?

Most of the commonly prescribed types of HRT for women going through the menopause combine daily estrogen with a 10- to 12-day course of progestogen, which results in a monthly withdrawal bleed, similar to a period. But you can take both progestogen and estrogen daily (continuous combined HRT) which should relieve your symptoms without a period.

Tibolone is a single daily tablet that combines the properties of estrogen and progestogen.

These methods are most suitable for women starting HRT several years after the menopause. They are not suitable for younger women because irregular bleeding is a common side effect.

Does HRT interfere with any other tablets that I take?

HRT is rarely affected by any other medication you might take. A few medicines interact with the way your liver breaks down hormones, which can make HRT less effective. This is more likely to happen if you take tablets for HRT than if you are using patches or implants. Medicines that might have this effect are some of those usually prescribed for epilepsy, such as phenytoin or carbamazepine. Some antibiotics have a similar effect. The herbal treatment St John's wort may also interact with HRT. Always check with your doctor if you have any doubts about what you are taking.

I've read that HRT increases the risk of thrombosis. Do I have to stop HRT when I'm flying?

HRT increases the chances of having a blood clot in the legs (a deep vein thrombosis or DVT) or lungs (a pulmonary embolism). This means that women on HRT are also at increased risk of having a blood clot on a long-haul plane flight, or in other situations where they are in prolonged cramped conditions. The standard advice about avoiding DVTs when flying is getting up and moving around regularly, drinking plenty of fluids and wearing support stockings during a flight. When seated in a plane, move your neck from side to side and up and down, and flex your ankles and wrists frequently – all to maintain good circulation.

I'm 62 and I've taken HRT for the last 10 years. I'd like to stop HRT. Can I just stop it immediately?

Stopping HRT abruptly can result in a return of the symptoms. To prevent this, HRT should be tailed off gradually over two to three months under the supervision of your doctor.

I'm 49 and started HRT six months ago. I was having terrible hot flushes before I started and my periods were all over the place. Although HRT has helped these symptoms, I'm not entirely happy with it. Whenever I take the progestogens each month I feel bloated and headachy – just like the terrible premenstrual symptoms I used to get with my periods. I'm not sure which is worse – stopping the HRT and getting the flushes back or continuing HRT and feeling so awful for two out of every four weeks. Is there a different type of HRT I could take?

Some women are very sensitive to the progestogen phase of sequential combined HRT, particularly if they experienced premenstrual symptoms in the past. Sometimes changing the type of progestogen, for example changing from norethisterone to dydrogesterone, can help. Otherwise, try changing to a sequential combined patch because non-oral routes contain lower doses of hormone compared with oral preparations. Progestogenic side effects are also less likely to occur with continuous combined HRT – partly because the dose of progestogen is lower when taken daily, and partly because continuous progestogen seems to cause fewer side effects than cycles of progestogen. Alternatively, consider the progestogen-containing intrauterine system. Some women favour natural progesterone available on prescription as vaginal gels, pessaries or rectal suppositories, but drowsiness is a common problem.

Glossary

Amenorrhoea: the absence of menstrual bleeding.

Bartholin's glands: small mucus-secreting glands situated one each side of the vaginal opening.

Climacteric: the transition through the menopause.

COC: the combined oral contraceptive pill.

Continuous combined HRT: a regimen of HRT involving daily estrogen and daily progestogen. This 'period'-free regimen is particularly suitable for women after the menopause.

DXA: dual-energy X-ray absorptiometry – a machine that uses minute doses of X-rays to measure the bone mineral density of the skeleton.

Down's syndrome: a condition characterised by a variety of physical abnormalities present at birth including moderate-to-severe mental handicap or learning disability.

Endometrium: the lining of the uterus, which thickens in response to estrogen.

Estrogen: a hormone produced by the ovaries. Deficiency of estrogen after the menopause is responsible for most of the symptoms associated with the menopause.

Follicle-stimulating hormone (FSH): a hormone produced by the pituitary gland in the brain. In a female it stimulates the growth of the follicle in the ovary.

HRT: hormone replacement therapy.

HERS: the Heart and (O)Estrogen/ Progestogen Replacement Study (HERS 1998). The HERS was designed to look at the effect of HRT on the rate of recurrent heart problems in women who already had heart disease.

IUS: the intrauterine system, a device containing a rod of progestogen that is inserted into the uterus to provide contraception and reduce menstrual bleeding. It can also be used to provide the progestogen component of HRT.

Licensed medication: when pharmaceutical companies develop new drugs, they undertake studies to assess safety and efficacy for the indication for which they developed the drug specifically. Once approved by the regulatory authorities, the drug can then be prescribed for this 'licensed' indication. However, once the drug has become widely used, it may be found to be safe and effective for a different condition. Doctors may prescribe the drug for this different condition, provided that the patient is aware that the regulatory authorities have not approved the drug for this different indication.

Most doctors will prescribe drugs 'off-licence' only if there is a specialist body that supports the use of the drug in that way. An example is the levonorgestrel intrauterine system (Mirena). In the UK, its licensed indication is for contraception and treatment of heavy periods. However, doctors have also found that it can safely and effectively be used as the progestogen component of HRT. Hence it is often prescribed 'off-licence' for this indication.

Long-cycle HRT: a regimen of HRT involving daily estrogen and a course of progestogen every three months. This results in four withdrawal bleeds every year.

Luteinising hormone (LH): a hormone produced by the pituitary gland that stimulates development of the corpus luteum in the ovaries.

Menopause: the stage of a woman's life when she has her last menstrual period.

Mini-pill: a popular name for the progestogen-only contraceptive pill.

MPA: medroxyprogesterone acetate – a type of progestogen used in HRT and for contraception.

Osteoporosis: a general term for describing any disease process that results in a reduction in the mass of bone per unit of volume. As a result bones are more fragile.

Ovulation: the periodic ripening and rupture of the mature follicle that discharges the ovum from the ovary into the fallopian tube.

Perimenopause: commonly used to mean the time between irregular periods and hot flushes starting and the years after the last menstrual period. Also called the menopause transition.

Phytoestrogen: plant-derived compounds with the properties of estrogen. Typically found in soy and red clover.

Placebo: a treatment containing no active ingredients given to a person participating in a clinical trial in order to assess the performance of an active treatment.

Placebo effect: a measurable improvement in health in a person given placebo.

Postmenopause: the time following a woman's last menstrual period.

Premature menopause: the term given to a natural or surgical menopause before the age of 40. Women who have an untreated premature menopause are at greater risk of heart disease and osteoporosis compared with women whose menopause occurs within the normal timeframe.

Premenopause: the time from a woman's first to last menstrual period.

Progesterone: a hormone produced by the ovaries. Necessary to protect the thickening of the uterine lining (endometrium) in response to estrogen, which if unchecked can lead to cancer.

Progestogen: a synthetic form of progesterone.

Sequential combined: a regimen of HRT involving daily estrogen and a course of progestogen taken for two out of every four weeks. This results in 13 withdrawal bleeds a year.

SERM: selective estrogen receptor modulator. SERMs are a relatively new group of drugs that include raloxifene (Evista). These synthetic drugs have estrogen-like effects on bone, increasing bone mass and reducing the risk of spinal fractures.

SSRI: selective serotonin reuptake inhibitor. SSRIs are a group of drugs licensed for the treatment of depression and include fluoxetine (Prozac).

STEAR: selective tissue estrogenic activity regulator. STEARs are a relatively new group of drugs that includes tibolone (Livial). These synthetic drugs combine the properties of estrogen, progesterone and testosterone.

Testosterone: a hormone produced in the testes of the male and to a lesser extent in a part of the brain of both males and females.

Venous thrombosis: a blood clot in the veins, typically affecting the calves. Occasionally a blood clot from the veins can reach the lungs – a pulmonary embolus.

WHI: the Women's Health Initiative study between 1993 and 1998: a set of clinical trials and an observational study set up by the National Institutes of Health in the USA. It was designed to test the risks and benefits of postmenopausal hormone therapy, diet modification, and calcium and vitamin D supplements on heart disease, breast and colorectal cancer, and bone fractures in postmenopausal women. More than 160,000 women aged 50–79 were enrolled as WHI participants.

Withdrawal bleed: when a course of progestogen is stopped, the resultant drop in hormone causes the lining of the uterus to break down and be shed as a withdrawal bleed or 'period'.

Useful addresses

We have included the following organisations because, on preliminary investigation, they may be of use to the reader. However, we do not have first-hand experience of each organisation and so cannot guarantee the organisation's integrity. The reader must therefore exercise his or her own discretion and judgement when making further enquiries.

Benefit Enquiry Line
Tel: 0800 882200 (Mon–Fri 8am–6pm)
Textphone: 0800 243355
Website: www.gov.uk/benefit-enquiry-line

Government agency giving information and advice on sickness and disability benefits for people with disabilities and their carers.

Macmillan Cancer Support
89 Albert Embankment
London SE1 7UQ
Helpline: 0808 808 0000
Tel: 020 7840 7840
Website: www.macmillan.org.uk

Provide quality-assured, up-to-date cancer information, written by specialists, for patients, relatives and carers.

Migraine Action
4th Floor, 27 East Street
Leicester LE1 6NB
Tel/helpline: 0116 275 8317 (Mon–Fri 10am–4pm)
Website: www.migraine.org.uk

Supports research, offers information on the understanding and treatment of migraine. Has dedicated websites for young migraineurs and a web forum.

The Migraine Trust
52–53 Russell Square
London WC1B 4HP
Tel: 020 7631 6970
Website: www.migrainetrust.org

Offers information, advice and training to migraine sufferers and their families. Has a support network, funds research and runs conferences on migraine.

fpa (Family Planning Association)
50 Featherstone Street
London EC1Y 8QU

Tel: 020 7608 5240
Helpline: 0845 122 8690 (Mon–Thurs 9am–3pm,
Fri 9am–midday)
Website: www.fpa.org.uk

Offers telephone advice on above helpline on
contraception and sexual health. Appointment needed
to view their reference library. Has a useful source of
up-to-date information about other services and
organisations relating to men's and women's health.

Institute for Complementary and Natural Medicine
Can-Mezzanine, 32–36 Loman Street
London SE1 0EH
Tel: 020 7922 7980
Website: www.i-c-m.org.uk

A registered charity formed as umbrella for complementary
medicine groups. Offers information, British register of
accredited practitioners and recommends approved training courses. An SAE requested with two first-class stamps.

**National Institute for Health and Clinical
Excellence (NICE)**
1st Floor, 10 Spring Gardens
London SW1A 2BU
Tel: 0845 003 7784
Website: www.nice.org.uk

Provides national guidance on the promotion of good
health and treatment of ill-health. Patient information
leaflets are available for each piece of guidance issued.

National Osteoporosis Society
Camerton
Bath, Somerset BA2 0PJ
Helpline: 0845 450 0230 (Mon–Fri 9am–5pm)
Tel: 0845 130 3076 (Mon–Thurs 9am–4.30pm,
Fri 9am–4pm)
Website: www.nos.org.uk

Provides information, advice and support for people with osteoporosis. Helpline staffed by specially trained nurses. Has local support groups.

NHS Direct
Tel: 0845 4647 (24 hours, 365 days a year)
Website: www.nhsdirect.nhs.uk

Offers confidential health-care advice, information and referral service. A good first port of call for any health advice.

NHS Smoking Helpline
Freephone: 0800 022 4332 (Mon–Fri 9am–8pm, Sat & Sun 11am–4pm)
Website: http://smokefree.nhs.uk

Have advice, help and encouragement on giving up smoking. Specialist advisers available to offer ongoing support to those who genuinely are trying to give up smoking. Can refer to local branches.

Patients' Association
PO Box 935
Harrow, Middlesex HA1 3YJ
Helpline: 0845 608 4455

Tel: 020 8423 9111
Website: www.patients-association.com

Provides advice on patients' rights, leaflets and a directory of self-help groups.

Quit (Smoking Quitlines)

20 Curtain Road
London EC2A 3NF
Helpline: 0800 002200 (Mon–Fri 9am–8pm, Sat, Sun 10am–4pm)
Tel: 020 7539 1700
Website: www.quit.org.uk

Offers individual advice on giving up smoking in English and Asian languages. Talks to schools on smoking and pregnancy and can refer to local support groups. Runs training courses for professionals.

Relate (the relationship people)

Premier House, Caroline Court, Lakeside
Doncaster DN4 5RA
Tel: 0300 100 1234
Website: www.relate.org.uk

Does not have counsellors on hand, but can refer you to one of 100 branches. Relate publications on health, sexual, self-esteem, depression, bereavement and re-marriage issues available via website or from bookshops and libraries.The address will be changing in the near future.

The Tavistock Centre for Couple Relationships

70 Warren Street

London W1T 5PB
Tel: 020 7380 1960
Website: www.tccr.org.uk

Runs counselling service for couples living or working in London.

Women's Health Concern
4–6 Eton Place, Marlow
Buckinghamshire SL7 2QA
Tel: 01628 890199
Website: www.womens-health-concern.org

Offers information, advice and counselling to women with gynaecological and hormonal problems. Publishes books and factsheets. Send an SAE for a current list of publications.

Websites
BBC
www.bbc.co.uk/health
A helpful website: easy to navigate and offers lots of useful advice and information. Also contains links to other related topics.

Healthtalkonline
www.healthtalkonline.org
Website of the DIPEx charity.

Menopause Matters
www.menopausematters.co.uk
Independent clinician-led website.

Patient UK
www.patient.co.uk

Useful information about medical conditions with clear diagrams for health professionals and patients.

The internet as a source of further information

After reading this book, you may feel that you would like further information on the subject. The internet is of course an excellent place to look and there are many websites with useful information about medical disorders, related charities and support groups.

For those who do not have a computer at home some bars and cafes offer facilities for accessing the internet. These are listed in the *Yellow Pages* under 'Internet Bars and Cafes' and 'Internet Providers'. Your local library offers a similar facility and has staff to help you find the information that you need.

It should always be remembered, however, that the internet is unregulated and anyone is free to set up a website and add information to it. Many websites offer impartial advice and information that has been compiled and checked by qualified medical professionals. Some, on the other hand, are run by commercial organisations with the purpose of promoting their own products. Others still are run by pressure groups, some of which will provide carefully assessed and accurate information whereas others may be suggesting medications or treatments that are not supported by the medical and scientific community.

Unless you know the address of the website you want to visit – for example, www.familydoctor.co.uk – you may find the following guidelines useful when searching the internet for information.

Search engines and other searchable sites

Google (www.google.co.uk) is the most popular search engine used in the UK, followed by Yahoo! (http://uk.yahoo.com) and MSN (www.msn.co.uk). Also popular are the search engines provided by Internet Service Providers such as TalkTalk and other sites such as the BBC site (www.bbc.co.uk).

In addition to the search engines that index the whole web, there are also medical sites with search facilities, which act almost like mini-search engines, but cover only medical topics or even a particular area of medicine. Again, it is wise to look at who is responsible for compiling the information offered to ensure that it is impartial and medically accurate. The NHS Direct site (www.nhsdirect.nhs.uk) is an example of a searchable medical site.

Links to many British medical charities can be found at the Association of Medical Research Charities' website (www.amrc.org.uk) and at Charity Choice (www.charitychoice.co.uk).

Search phrases

Be specific when entering a search phrase. Searching for information on 'cancer' will return results for many different types of cancer as well as on cancer in general. You may even find sites offering astrological information. More useful results will be returned by using search phrases such as 'lung cancer' and 'treatments for lung cancer'. Both Google and Yahoo! offer an advanced search option that includes the ability to search for the exact phrase; enclosing the search phrase in quotes, that is, 'treatments for lung cancer', will have the same effect. Limiting a search to an exact phrase reduces the number of results returned but it is best to refine a search to an exact match only if you are not getting useful results with a normal search. Adding 'UK' to your search term will bring up mainly British sites, so a good phrase might be 'lung cancer' UK (don't include UK within the quotes).

Always remember the internet is international and unregulated. It holds a wealth of valuable information but individual sites may be biased, out of date or just plain wrong. Family Doctor Publications accepts no responsibility for the content of links published in this series.

Index

abdominal pains, as side effect of HRT 109
acne, as side effect of HRT 109
Actonel (risedronate) 55, 57
acupuncture 32
Adcal preparations 56
age at menopause 1
air travel, venous thrombosis risk 145–6
alcohol consumption 22, 28–9, 50
alendronate sodium (Fosamax) 55, 57
17-alpha-dihydroequilin 75
amenorrhoea 148
 – osteoporosis risk 52–3
Angeliq 92–3
anorexia nervosa, osteoporosis risk 53
antibiotics, interaction with HRT 145
anxiety 7
aromatherapy 32
arthritis
 – effects of HRT 58–9

 – *see also* rheumatoid arthritis
artificial tears 21
aspirin, interaction with ginseng 125
Association of Medical Research Charities 161
atherosclerosis 22, 71
athletes, osteoporosis risk 53

backache, as side effect of HRT 109
barrier methods of contraception 133
Bartholin's glands 148
bathing, skin patches 79
BBC website 159
bed rest, osteoporosis risk 52
Bedol 94
Benefit Enquiry Line 154
biofeedback 32
bisphosphonates 55, 57, 143
black cohosh 124
bladder weakness 8
 – self-help 17–18

bleeding
- during continuous combined HRT 99–100
- investigation of 110–14
- as side effect of HRT 110
- undiagnosed, avoidance of HRT 121
- when to seek medical advice 34, 98, 102

bloating, as side effect of HRT 108

blood clots 61
- risk from HRT 40, 43
- see also venous thrombosis

blood tests
- before starting HRT 141–2
- diagnosis of the menopause 10–11

body mass index (BMI) 29, 30
- effect on breast cancer risk 65
- high, risks 51
- low, osteoporosis risk 51

bone, effects of osteoporosis 47, 49

bone density
- effectiveness of prescribed treatments 88
- effect of raloxifene 143–4
- see also osteoporosis

bone density measurement 49, 50, 143

bone loss see osteoporosis

Bonefos (sodium clodronate) 55, 57

Bonviva (ibandronate) 55, 57

bowel cancer 12

brain haemorrhages 70

breast cancer 12, 61
- non-HRT risk factors 64–6
- protective effect of raloxifene 143–4
- risk from HRT 37, 40, 43, 62–4, 74, 104, 137
- risk from tibolone 88, 90

breast cancer patients, use of HRT 66, 119–20

breast-feeding, effect on breast cancer risk 65

breast screening 32

breast tenderness, as side effect of HRT 108, 109

breasts
- lumps 32, 34, 140
- benign, taking HRT 118
- self-awareness 32
- self-examination 140
- skin changes 34

Cacit preparations 56

caffeine, link to osteoporosis 52

Calceos 56

Calcichew preparations 56

calcitonin (Miacalcic) 57, 58

calcitriol 57

calcium intake 26, 52
- dietary sources of calcium 27

calcium supplements 27–8
- preparations available 56

Calfovit D₃ 56

cancer treatment, premature menopause 1, 45

carbamazepine, interaction with HRT 145

Cerazette 131

cervical cancer, HRT 117

cervical screening 32–3

'change of life' 1
- see also menopause

Charity Choice 161

chemotherapy, premature
      menopause 1, 45
children, diet and exercise 23
cholecalciferol 57
  – see also vitamin D
    supplements
cholecystitis risk, effect of
      HRT 43
cholesterol levels
  – effect of raloxifene 143–4
  – high, using HRT 117
Clasteon (sodium clodronate)
      57
climacteric 1, 148
  – see also menopause
Climagest 92–3
Climanor
      (medroxyprogesterone
      acetate) 87
Climaval 94
Climesse 92–3
clinical trials of HRT 38–40
Clinorette 92–3
clonidine, for hot flushes 127
coeliac disease
  – osteoporosis risk 53
  – using HRT 117
coitus interruptus
      (withdrawal method)
      134
colorectal cancer risk, effect
      of HRT 40, 43, 59, 137
combined oral contraceptive
      130
  – for hot flushes 127
complementary treatments
      31–2
  – Institute for
    Complementary Medicine
    156
concentration problems 9–10
condoms 133

conjugated equine estrogens
      36, 41
  – combination with
    progestogens 92–3
  – risk of breast cancer 74
  – unopposed estrogen
    preparations 94
continuous combined HRT
      99–101, 148
contraception 136
  – barrier methods 133
  – coitus interruptus 134
  – combined hormonal
    contraceptives 130
  – copper intrauterine
    devices 133
  – Family Planning
    Association 155–6
  – fertility awareness 134
  – how long to continue
    using it 5
  – and HRT 135
  – levonorgestrel
    intrauterine system
    (Mirena) 132
  – need for 129–30
  – progestogen-only
    methods 130–2
  – spermicides 134
  – sterilisation 133
  – vaginal sponge 133–4
  – when you can stop using
    it 134, 135
contraceptive patch 130
copper intrauterine devices
      133
Crinone 87
Crohn's disease, HRT 117
Cushing's disease,
      osteoporosis risk 53
cyclical (sequential combined)
      HRT 97–9

Cyclo-Progynova 92–3
cystitis, self-help 18, 20

dairy products, calcium
content 26, 27
Deca-Durabolin (nandrolone)
57
deep vein thrombosis 67
– risk from flying 145–6
denosumab (Prolia) 57
Depo-Provera 131
depression 7, 9–10, 141
– self-help 22
– as side effect of HRT 109
– SSRIs 126–7
Desunin 57
diabetes, using HRT 117
diabetes risk, effect of HRT
43
diagnosis of the menopause
10–11
diaphragms 133
Didronel (etidronate sodium)
55, 57
dienoestrol 75
diet
– alcohol consumption
28–9
– calcium intake 26
– iron intake 15
– natural estrogens 26
– supplements 27–8
– vitamin D intake 26–7
– weight control 29
dieting, osteoporosis risk 53
DMPA (depot
medroxyprogesterone
acetate) 131
dong quai 123, 124
'dowager's hump' 49
Down's syndrome 129,
148–9

drospirenone, in combined
HRT preparations 92–3
DXA (dual-energy X-ray
absorptiometry) 49,
50, 148
dydrogesterone, in combined
HRT preparations 92–3

Efexor (venlafaxine) 126–7
Elleste Duet preparations
92–3
Elleste Solo preparations 94
emotional symptoms 9–10
– self-help 22
– see also depression
endometrial biopsy 111–13,
114
endometrial cancer 61
– risk from estrogen
therapy 36–7, 43, 73
endometrial cancer patients,
use of HRT 120
endometriosis
– benefits of progestogens
97
– HRT 118
– treatment, osteoporosis
risk 53
endometrium 149
– changes during menstrual
cycle 2
epilepsy, using HRT 117, 145
equilin 75
Estraderm preparations 94
estradiol 41, 63, 75
– combination with
progestogens 92–3
– local preparations 95
– unopposed estrogen
preparations 94
Estradot 94
Estring 95

estriol 75
- local preparations 95
estrogen 149
- changes during menstrual cycle 2, 3, 4
- changes over a lifetime 3
- continuous treatment 101
- cyclical treatment 101
- natural estrogens 26
- side effects 108
- synthetic 36
estrogen dose 102
estrogen levels, measurement before implant insertion 85
estrogen preparations 75-6
- gels 81-2
- implants 82-3
- oral tablets 77-8
- skin patches 79-80
- vaginal creams, pessaries and tablets 85-6, 95
estrone 75
ethinylestradiol 75
etidronate sodium (Didronel) 55, 57
evening primrose oil 108, 123, 124-5
Evista (raloxifene) 57, 58, 144
Evorel preparations 92-3, 94
exercise 16
- benefits 14, 23-4
- as a daily routine 25
- in prevention of osteoporosis 52
eyes, dryness 9
- self-help 21

factor V Leiden 68
falls, risk reduction 24

family difficulties 10
family history
- of breast cancer 65-6
- of osteoporosis 51-2
- of venous thrombosis 121
Family Planning Association (fpa) 155-6
Femidom 133
Femoston preparations 92-3
FemSeven preparations 92-3, 94
fertility awareness 134
fibroids 119
fish consumption 26-7
fish oil supplements 16
fluid intake 21
fluid retention 108, 109
fluoxetine (Prozac) 126-7
flushes see hot flushes
follicle-stimulating hormone (FSH) 149
- blood tests 10
Forsteo (teriparatide) 57, 58
Fosamax (alendronate sodium) 55, 57
Fosavance 55, 57
fracture risk, effect of HRT 43
fractures 23, 48
- family history of 51-2
- as risk factor for osteoporosis 53
- see also osteoporosis
Fultium-D$_3$ 57

gabapentin 127
gallstones, using HRT 119
gel HRT 64, 76, 81-2
- advantages and disadvantages 90
ginseng 123, 125
glucosamine 16

gymnasts, osteoporosis risk 53
Gynest 95

hair
– changes after the menopause 9
– dryness, self-help 20–1
headaches 7
– self-help 16
– as side effect of HRT 115
Healthtalkonline 159
'healthy user effect', HRT 37
Heart and Estrogen/Progestogen Replacement Study (HERS) 38–9, 149
heart attack patients, use of HRT 121
heart disease 12
– atherosclerosis 71
– non-HRT risk factors 72
– prevention
– lifestyle changes 22–3
– value of exercise 23–5
– what it is 22
heart disease risk
– effect of alcohol consumption 28, 29
– effect of HRT 37–40, 42, 43, 68–9, 72–3, 74, 137
heart valve disease, using HRT 118
heavy periods 15
height, loss of 49, 143
help, where to find it
– searching the internet 160–2
– useful addresses 154–9
– websites 159–60
herbalism 32

high blood pressure, HRT 117
hip fractures 23, 48
– see also osteoporosis
homeopathy 32
hormone replacement therapy (HRT) 44, 60, 137–9
– advantages and disadvantages of different types 90–1
– availability 75
– for breast cancer patients 66
– choices flowchart 98
– continuous combined 99–101
– continuous estrogen 101
– and contraception 135
– cyclical estrogen 101
– doses of estrogen and progestogen 102
– drug interactions 145
– effect on colorectal cancer risk 59
– effects on arthritis 58–9
– estrogen preparations 75–6
– local 95
– estrogen/progestogen combinations 92–3
– how long it has been available 35–6
– how long to take it for 104–5
– after hysterectomy 101
– importance of progesterone 97
– indications for use 35
– for menopausal symptoms 46
– methods of administration 76

– gels 81–2
– implants 82–5
– oral tablets 77–9
– skin patches 79–81
– vaginal (local) estrogen 85–6
– osteoporosis prevention 47
– osteoporosis treatment 49
– for premature menopause 45–6
– progesterone preparations 86–7
– progestogen preparations 76, 77
– importance 97
– raloxifene (Evista) 58
– risks 61, 74, 144
– breast cancer 62–4
– endometrial cancer 73
– heart attacks and strokes 68–9, 72–3
– ovarian cancer 73
– venous thrombosis 66–8
– risks versus benefits 36–8, 41–3
– recent studies 38–40
– sequential combined (cyclical) 97–9
– side effects 79, 108–10, 116, 146–7
– bleeding 110
– headaches 115
– weight gain 115
– stopping treatment 105–6, 107, 146
– tibolone (Livial) 88, 95
– unopposed estrogen preparations 94
– for vaginal symptoms only 101–2

– what it is 35
– when to start treatment 104
– who can take it 117–18
– who should be cautious 118–19
– who should not take it 119–21
Hormonin 94
hot flushes 5–6
– combined oral contraceptives 127
– effect of HRT 46
– effectiveness of different types of HRT 88
– non-hormonal prescriptions 126–7
– non-prescription remedies 123–6
– progestogens 128
– self-help 14–15
housebound people, osteoporosis risk 53
HRT see hormone replacement therapy
hydroxyethylcellulose 21
hypromellose 21
hysterectomy
– early menopause 45
– HRT 101
hysteroscopy 113–14

ibandronate (Bonviva) 55, 57
Implanon 132
implant contraception 132
76
– advantages 83
– disadvantages 83–5, 91
– estrogen 82–3
– method of insertion 84
– stopping treatment 106
– testosterone 83

incontinence of urine 8
– self-help 17–18, 19
Indivina 92–3
infections, urinary 8–9
– self-help 18, 20
inflammatory bowel disease, osteoporosis risk 53
injectable contraception 131
Institute for Complementary Medicine 156
intercourse, painful 8
intrauterine devices (IUDs) 133
intrauterine system (IUS) 149
– see also levonorgestrel intrauterine system (Mirena)
iron intake 15
irregular periods 4, 5
– self-help 15
isoflavones 123, 124

jaundice, use of HRT 120
jaw osteonecrosis 55
joint pains 7
– self-help 16

Kalcipos-D 56
Kegel exercises 18
kidney disease, HRT 117
Kliofem 92–3
Kliovance 92–3
KY jelly 17

leg cramps, as side effect of HRT 108
lethargy 9–10
levonorgestrel, in combined HRT preparations 92–3
levonorgestrel intrauterine system (Mirena) 86–7, 89, 132

– with continuous estrogen 100–1
– for fibroids 119
libido, loss of 8, 141
– self-help 17
– testosterone therapy 83
licensed medication 149–50
lifelong HRT 105
lifestyle changes
– in prevention of heart disease 22–3
– in prevention of osteoporosis 23
liquorice 123, 125
liver disease
– osteoporosis risk 53
– use of HRT 117, 120
Livial (tibolone) 88, 90–1, 95, 145
long-cycle HRT 98–9, 150
Loron (sodium clodronate) 55, 57
lubricating gels 16–17
lumps in breasts 32, 34, 140
– benign, using HRT 118
lung cancer risk, effect of HRT 43
luteinising hormone (LH) 150
– blood tests 10
– changes during menstrual cycle 2

malignant melanoma, using HRT 117
mammography screening 32
Macmillan Cancer Support 155
'matrix' skin patches 79
medical advice, when to seek it 34

medroxyprogesterone acetate (MPA) 150
– in combined HRT preparations 92–3
– Depo-Provera 131
– for hot flushes 128
– preparations available 87
megestrol acetate, for hot flushes 128
menopause
– adjusting to changes 4
– diagnosis 10–11
– premature 1
– what it is 1, 150
Menopause Matters website 159
menstrual cycle 2, 4
menstruation, early onset, effect on breast cancer risk 64
mestranol 75
Miacalcic (calcitonin) 57, 58
migraine 7
– self-help 16
– as side effect of HRT 115
– useful addresses 155
– using HRT 118
Migraine Action 155
Migraine Trust, The 155
Million Women Study 38
mini-pill 131, 150
Mirena intrauterine system 86–7, 89, 132
– with continuous estrogen 100–1
– for fibroids 119
miscarriage risk 129
missed tablets, HRT 79, 100
monoamine oxidase inhibitors (MAOIs), interaction with ginseng 125

mood swings, as side effect of HRT 109
MPA see medroxyprogesterone acetate
muscle pains 7
– self-help 16

nandrolone (Deca-Durabolin) 57
Natecal D₃ 56
National Institute for Health and Clinical Excellence (NICE) 156
National Osteoporosis Society 157
natural estrogens 26, 75
natural progesterone preparations 86, 123, 125–6, 147
nausea, as side effect of HRT 79, 108
NHS Direct 157
NHS Smoking Helpline 157
night sweats 5, 6
– effect of HRT 46
– effectiveness of different types of HRT 88
– self-help 14–15
nipple changes 32, 34
norethisterone
– in combined HRT preparations 92–3
– Noristerat 131
Novofem 92–3
Nuvelle Continuous 92–3

observational studies 38
Oestrogel 94
oestrogen see estrogen
'off-licence' use of medication 149–50

oophorectomy (removal of the ovaries) 45
oral contraceptives
– for hot flushes 127
– protection against osteoporosis 54
Ortho-Gynest 95
osteoarthritis, effect of HRT 58–9
osteonecrosis of the jaw 55
osteopathy 32
osteoporosis 46–7, 151
– diagnosis 49, 50
– National Osteoporosis Society 157
– prevention 105, 143
– by HRT 47
– lifestyle changes 23
– value of exercise 24–5
– protective factors 51, 54–5
– combined oral contraceptive 130
– risk factors 50–4
– alcohol consumption 28
– treatment 49, 57–8
– bisphosphonates 55
– what it is 23
otosclerosis, using HRT 119
ovarian cancer
– risk from HRT 61, 73
– using HRT 118
Ovestin 95
ovulation 151
– hormone changes 2, 4

painful periods 15
painkillers
– for headaches 16
– for joint and muscle pains 16
– for painful periods 15
palpitations 6
parity, relationship to osteoporosis risk 54–5
Parkinson's disease
– dry eyes 21
– HRT 118
paroxetine (Seroxat) 126–7
patch HRT see skin patches
Patient UK 159
Patients' Association 157–8
peak bone mass 23, 24
pelvic floor exercises 17–18, 19
perimenopause 151
period problems
– self-help 15
– when to seek medical advice 34
period-free HRT 78, 144–5
– continuous combined HRT 99–101
– preparations available 92–3
– tibolone (Livial) 88, 90–1
periods
– changes around the menopause 4, 5, 143
– during HRT 77, 78, 98, 110
– lack of, osteoporosis risk 52–3
phenytoin, interaction with HRT 145
physiotherapy 32
phytoestrogens 124, 151
pill see combined oral contraceptive; progestogen-only pill
placebo-controlled clinical trials 38
placebo effect 151

placebos 151
postmenopausal risks 11–12
postmenopause 151
pregnancy
– effect on breast cancer
risk 65
– protection against
osteoporosis 54–5
– while taking HRT 121
Premarin 94, 142
premature menopause 1,
45, 151
– effect on breast cancer
risk 64
– HRT 46, 60, 105, 107
– breast cancer risk 62
premenopause 152
premenstrual symptoms 7
– as side effect of HRT 109
Premique preparations 92–3,
142
Prempak-C 92–3
progesterone 77, 152
– blood tests 10
– changes during menstrual
cycle 2, 4
– natural progesterone
preparations 125–6
– preparations available
86–7
progestogen dose, HRT 102
progestogen-only
contraception 130–2
progestogen-only pill (POP)
131
progestogen preparations 76
progestogens 77, 152
– in endometriosis 118
– for hot flushes 128
– importance in HRT 97
– inclusion in HRT 37
– oral tablets 78

– side effects 109–10,
146–7
– use with local vaginal
estrogens 102
Progynova preparations 94
Prolia (denosumab) 57
Protelos (strontium ranelate)
57, 58
Provera (medroxyprogesterone
acetate) 87
Prozac (fluoxetine) 126–7
pulmonary embolism 67
– risk from flying 145–6

Quit (smoking Quitlines) 158

racial origins, relationship to
osteoporosis risk 54
radiotherapy, premature
menopause 1, 45
raloxifene (Evista) 57, 58,
143–4
red clover, isoflavones 124
Relate 158
relaxation, in management of
hot flushes 15
Replens 17
rheumatoid arthritis
– effect of HRT 58–9
– osteoporosis risk 53
– using HRT 118
risedronate (Actonel) 55, 57
– preparations available 57
Rocaltrol 57

'safe period' method of
contraception 134
Sandocal preparations 56
Sandrena 94
screening
– for breast cancer 32
– cervical 32–3

Senselle 17
sequential combined (cyclical) HRT 97–9, 152
SERMs (selective estrogen receptor modulators) 58, 143–4, 152
Seroxat (paroxetine) 126–7
sexual problems 8, 141
– self-help 16–17
side effects of HRT 79, 108–10, 116, 146–7
– bleeding 110
– headaches 115
– weight gain 115
Sjögren's syndrome 21
Skelid (tiludronic acid) 55, 57
skin
– changes over breasts 34
– dryness 9, 21
skin patches 64, 76
– absorption of hormones 81
– advantages 80, 90
– disadvantages 80–1, 90
– estrogen 79–80
– estrogen/progestogen combinations 80
– site of application 79
sleep disturbance 7
– self-help 15
smear tests 32–3
smoking, risks 31, 51
smoking cessation
– benefits 15
– NHS Smoking Helpline 157
– Quit (smoking Quitlines) 158
sodium clodronate (Bonefos, Clasteon, Loron) 55, 57

soya bean products, natural estrogens 26, 124
speculum examinations 33
spermicides 134
spinal (vertebral) fractures 23
– see also osteoporosis
SSRIs (selective serotonin reuptake inhibitors) 152
– for hot flushes 126–7
St John's wort, interaction with HRT 145
STEARs (selective tissue estrogenic activity regulators) 88, 95, 152
sterilisation 133
steroid treatment, osteoporosis risk 54
stomach upset, as side effect of HRT 108
stress incontinence 8
– self-help 17–18
stroke patients, use of HRT 121
stroke risk
– effect of alcohol consumption 29
– effect of HRT 37, 40, 69, 72–3, 137
strokes 12, 22
– causes 70
strontium ranelate (Protelos) 57, 58
subarachnoid haemorrhage 70
sunbathing, skin patches 80
sunlight, lack of, osteoporosis risk 53
surgery, prevention of blood clots 68

sweats *see* night sweats
swimming
 – exercise value 25
 – skin patches 79
symptoms of the menopause
  4, 6, 13, 143
 – dry eyes 9
 – dry skin and hair 9
 – effect of HRT 46
 – effectiveness of different
   types of HRT 88
 – emotional symptoms
   9–10
 – headaches 7
 – hot flushes and night
   sweats 5–6
 – irregular periods 5
 – joint and muscle pains 7
 – loss of libido 8
 – non-hormonal symptoms
   10
 – painful intercourse 8
 – self-help 14–22
 – sleep disturbance 7
 – urinary symptoms 8–9
 – vaginal dryness 16–17
 – weight gain 9
synthetic estrogens 75, 76
systemic HRT 76

tablets, HRT 77–9
 – advantages and
   disadvantages 90
tachyphylaxis 84
Tavistock Centre for Couple
  Relationships 158–9
tears, artificial 21
teriparatide (Forsteo) 57,
  58
testosterone 152
testosterone implants 83
thrombophilia 121

thrombosis, as cause of
  strokes 70
thyroid diseases
 – dry eyes 21
 – HRT 118
 – osteoporosis risk 53
tibolone (Livial) 88, 90–1,
  95, 145
tiludronic acid (Skelid) 55,
  57
tiredness 9–10, 141
tofu, natural estrogens 26
transvaginal ultrasound scans
  (TVS) 111, 114
Tridestra 92–3
Trisequens 92–3

ultrasound scans,
  transvaginal (TVS) 111,
  114
units of alcohol 28, 29
urinary infections, self-help
  18, 20
urinary symptoms 8–9
 – self-help 17–20
uterus, cancer of *see*
  endometrial cancer
uterus lining *see*
  endometrium
Utrogestan 87

Vagifem 95
vagina, changes after the
  menopause 8
vaginal application of
  hormones 76
 – advantages and
   disadvantages 91
 – estrogen 85–6
vaginal cones 18, 19
vaginal ring 76
 – contraceptive 130

vaginal sponge 133–4
vaginal symptoms
 – effect of HRT 46
 – effectiveness of different
 types of HRT 88
 – local estrogen therapy
 101–2
 – self-help 16–17
vasectomy 133
venlafaxine (Efexor) 126–7
venous thrombosis 66–8,
 74, 153
 – family history 121
 – risk from flying 145–6
 – risk from raloxifene 144
vertebral (spinal) fractures
 23
 – see also osteoporosis
vitamin A deficiency, dry eyes
 21
vitamin D analogue
 (Rocaltrol) 57
vitamin D intake 26–7
vitamin D production,
 importance of sunlight
 exposure 53
vitamin D supplements 27–8
 – preparations available
 56, 57
vitamin E 123, 125

walking, exercise value 25
warfarin, interaction with
 ginseng 125
weight-bearing exercise 25
weight control 29
 – what you should weigh
 30
weight gain 9, 21–2
 – as side effect of HRT 115
weight reduction, benefits
 15, 16, 17
withdrawal bleeds 77, 78,
 98, 110, 144, 153
withdrawal method of
 contraception (coitus
 interruptus) 134
Women's Health Concern
 159
Women's Health Initiative
 (WHI) study 38, 39–40,
 69, 72, 153
 – criticisms 41
wrist fractures 48
 – see also osteoporosis

Zumenon 94

Your pages

We have included the following pages because they may help you manage your illness or condition and its treatment.

Before an appointment with a health professional, it can be useful to write down a short list of questions of things that you do not understand, so that you can make sure that you do not forget anything.

Some of the sections may not be relevant to your circumstances.

We are always pleased to receive constructive criticism or suggestions about how to improve the books. You can contact us at:

Email: familydoctor@btinternet.com
Letter: Family Doctor Publications
         PO Box 4664
         Poole
         BH15 1NN

Thank you

Health-care contact details

Name:

Job title:

Place of work:

Tel:

Name:

Job title:

Place of work:

Tel:

Name:

Job title:

Place of work:

Tel:

Name:

Job title:

Place of work:

Tel:

**Significant past health events – illnesses/
operations/investigations/treatments**

Event	Month	Year	Age (at time)

Appointments for health care

Name:

Place:

Date:

Time:

Tel:

Name:

Place:

Date:

Time:

Tel:

Name:

Place:

Date:

Time:

Tel:

Name:

Place:

Date:

Time:

Tel:

Appointments for health care

Name:

Place:

Date:

Time:

Tel:

Name:

Place:

Date:

Time:

Tel:

Name:

Place:

Date:

Time:

Tel:

Name:

Place:

Date:

Time:

Tel:

Current medication(s) prescribed by your doctor

Medicine name:

Purpose:

Frequency & dose:

Start date:

End date:

Medicine name:

Purpose:

Frequency & dose:

Start date:

End date:

Medicine name:

Purpose:

Frequency & dose:

Start date:

End date:

Medicine name:

Purpose:

Frequency & dose:

Start date:

End date:

Other medicines/supplements you are taking, not prescribed by your doctor

Medicine/treatment:

Purpose:

Frequency & dose:

Start date:

End date:

Medicine/treatment:

Purpose:

Frequency & dose:

Start date:

End date:

Medicine/treatment:

Purpose:

Frequency & dose:

Start date:

End date:

Medicine/treatment:

Purpose:

Frequency & dose:

Start date:

End date:

Questions to ask at appointments

(Note: do bear in mind that doctors work under great time
pressure, so long lists may not be helpful for either of you)

Questions to ask at appointments
(Note: do bear in mind that doctors work under great time
pressure, so long lists may not be helpful for either of you)

Notes

Notes

Notes